I0477087

Practical Psoriasis Management

MICHAEL E. FARHANGIAN

KATHRYN L. ANDERSON

STEVEN R. FELDMAN

Copyright © 2015 Steven R. Feldman
All rights reserved.
ISBN: 151514769X
ISBN-13: +89-1515147695

CONTENTS

ACKNOWLEDGMENTS

We would like to extend a very special thank you to all of the faculty at the Wake Forest Department of Dermatology for their support.

We would also like to thank all of those who contributed to this book, without their wonderful contributions this book would have been no more than an idea.

Michael E. Farhangian

Kathryn L. Anderson

Steven R. Feldman

Chapter 1: Introduction to Practical Psoriasis Management

Michael E. Farhangian

How to use this book

The purpose of this book is to aid practitioners to effectively treat psoriasis in the majority of patients. Since psoriasis is a complex disease and psychosocial factors play a large role, we emphasize the importance of adherence to treatment and providing support in addition to describing treatment modalities.

The management of psoriasis is usually relatively straightforward, and the choice of therapy can be made in a structured way as shown in Figure 1. This book provides detailed information on use of the common psoriasis treatments. We have added checklists as well as tips and tricks throughout this book to help simplify the process.

Introduction to psoriasis

Psoriasis is an inflammatory disease that causes skin to become itchy, scaly and red. Psoriasis can happen in almost any place on the body, but the most common places are the scalp, elbows and knees. Examination of the gluteal cleft and the nails can also be helpful by identifying signs of psoriasis that confirm the diagnosis. Psoriasis is quite common; approximately 2-3% of people in the United States suffer from psoriasis in some form. Although it can start at any age, psoriasis most commonly manifests in people who are aged 15-30, it can, but is rare, to start in patients under the age of 10.

Types of Psoriasis

There are different forms of psoriasis, with plaque psoriasis being the most common subtype, affecting 90% of patients. Although patients with plaque psoriasis generally suffer with it for life, patients with acute guttate psoriasis may have a long remission after treatment. While all psoriasis has microscopic pustules histologically, when the pustules are large enough to see, the psoriasis is called pustular psoriasis. Treatment for most forms of psoriasis is the same, but pustular and other forms of very inflamed psoriasis are managed acutely a little differently, avoiding irritating treatments (tar, ultraviolet light) that might make the inflammation worse.

Determining the extent of the patient's disease is a key step in planning treatment for the patient (Table 1). For instance, patients with limited disease (often called "mild-to-moderate" disease) are those who feel they have few enough spots that they can realistically put topicals on all their spots; these are generally people with psoriasis affecting less than 10% of body surface area. Patients with more extensive disease (those who have so much involvement that they cannot realistically treat all their spots with topicals) require photo or systemic treatment (Table 2).

Table 1. Psoriasis overview

Common Subtypes	Appearance and location	Treatment
Plaque	Salmon colored plaques with silvery scale Elbows, knees, scalp, lower buttocks area, genitals	Phototherapy Topical and systemic medications
Inverse	Minimal scaling Located in skin folds: armpit, neck, inguinal area	Topical medications
Guttate	Small drop-like lesions Upper trunk and extremities	Spontaneous remission in children Phototherapy and topical treatment
Erythrodermic	Very red with superficial scaling Generalized location	Systemic medications
Pustular	Small, raised lesions filled with pus Can be generalized or on hands and feet	Systemic medications

Table 2. Treatment options for psoriasis

Mild Disease	More Severe Disease
Topical corticosteroids	Methotrexate
Topical vitamin D analogs	Acitretin
Combination vitamin D and topical steroids	Cyclosporine
Topical calcineurin inhibitors	Apremilast
Localized phototherapy	Biologics: Adalimumab, etanercept, ustekinumab, secukinumab For psoriatic arthritis only: Certolizumab and golimumab
Less commonly used treatments: topical anthralin, salicylic acid, and coal tar	Phototherapy (with or without acitretin) and laser
	Combination with topical and/or systemic treatments

Psoriasis Triggers and Contributors

Many factors may trigger psoriasis in previously healthy patients or may worsen psoriasis in someone who already has a low level of disease. Like many diseases, there is a strong genetic component of psoriasis, which predisposes individuals with a family history to have a higher risk of developing it. People might also find that their psoriasis started after beginning a certain medication such as lithium, or after an infection such as bacterial pharyngitis. Trauma to the skin may also precipitate psoriasis lesions, known as the Koebner phenomenon.

There are also lifestyle choices that may have an impact on psoriasis. People who are obese tend to have more severe psoriasis, though obesity may not have an impact on the onset of the disease. Conversely, smoking may lead to an increased risk of manifesting the disease. Like obese people, smokers also tend to suffer from more severe disease. Stress can also lead to the manifestation of psoriasis in some patients as well as the exacerbation of it. Whether these associations are real or not, controlling obesity, avoiding smoking and reducing stress are prudent measures.

Diagnosing Psoriasis

The diagnosis of psoriasis can many times be made based on its location and appearance (Table 1). Lesions of psoriasis can vary in size, but in general they are raised lesions that are thickened, red, and scaly. Patients with psoriasis usually have lesions on both the left and right sides of their body. Another characteristic finding of psoriasis is bleeding when the scales of psoriasis are picked off, called the Auspitz sign. In cases where the diagnosis of psoriasis is not clear, a biopsy or referral to specialist might be indicated.

Approach to Treating Psoriasis

The treatment of psoriasis with medication should be individualized to the patient. Those with more mild, localized psoriasis may be treated with topical treatment alone, whereas patients with more generalized, severe disease usually require systemic treatments (Figure 1).

Interpreting drug efficacy

The efficacy of systemic treatments for psoriasis in clinical trials is generally measured using the Psoriasis Area and Severity Index (PASI) score, which rates the psoriasis severity on the basis of induration, scaliness and erythema as well as body surface area involvement. Higher PASI scores indicate worse disease; any PASI score greater than 12 is severe disease.

Psoriasis studies frequently assess the percentage of patients who achieve success with the treatment. In studies of systemic psoriasis treatments, a 75% improvement in PASI score is considered success. The term PASI75 is used to indicate the percentage of patients who achieve a 75% improvement in PASI score. We will provide the PASI75 scores for systemic psoriasis treatments in order to compare the relative efficacy of these treatments.

Figure 1. Psoriasis Treatment Flowchart

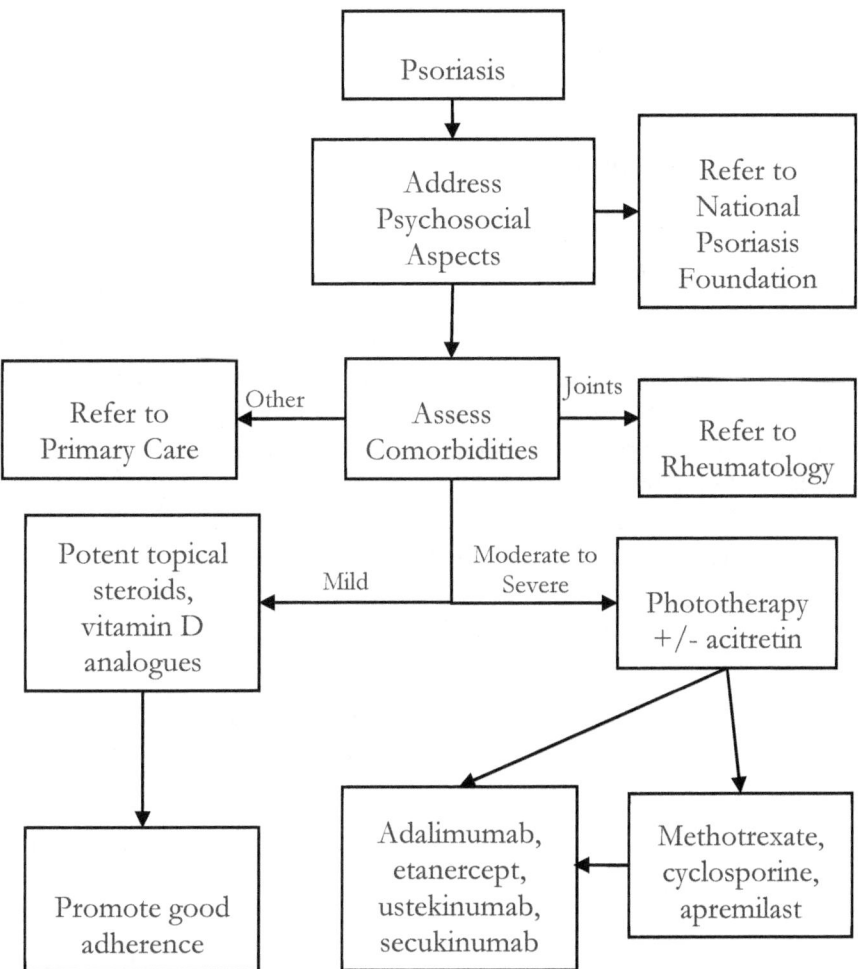

The above figure goes through a simplified algorithm for treating psoriasis. Prior to providing treatment, it is essential to ensure that patients are provided with the support they need, since psoriasis is a lifelong disease that can have a very large psychological impact on patients. Having patients become part of the National Psoriasis Foundation can make them feel supported. Also, since psoriasis is a systemic disease that impacts the skin and since systemic medications can exacerbate certain medical conditions, patients should be treated for their comorbid conditions.

The approach to treating psoriasis should be first to determine if patients have mild or more severe disease. Patients with mild disease can be managed with topical treatments (usually potent topical steroids and/or topical vitamin D) with an emphasis placed on good adherence to treatment. Those with more severe disease usually require treatment with systemic medications, with biologic medications generally being the most effective and least toxic (though phototherapy is well tolerated as well). However, in order for patients to qualify for treatment with biologics, they usually must fail other systemic medications such as methotrexate. A combination of topical medications can be used with systemic medications, with potent topical steroids playing a central role. Systemic treatments can also be used together, with methotrexate and biologics being a common combination.

Tips and Tricks

1. Keep in mind inverse psoriasis in patients with lesions in intertriginous areas

2. Biopsy and referral is rarely needed to diagnose and treat psoriasis

Table 2. Checklist

1.	Ask about any family history of psoriasis	
2.	Identify any possible triggers such as:	
	A. Smoking and inform them that quitting may help their psoriasis	
	B. Drugs including beta blockers, interferon, NSAIDs, ACE inhibitors,	
	C. Infections such as pharyngitis	
3.	Determine the extent of the patient's psoriasis (>10% body surface area is considered more severe)	
4.	Determine the subtype of psoriasis	

Chapter 2: Patient Resources and Education

Kathryn L. Anderson

Psoriasis is a chronic disease without a cure, and patients frequently feel overwhelmed and isolated when they receive the diagnosis. The first step in treatment is assuring the patient has reliable sources of psoriasis information and support. Patients often do not receive an adequate explanation of their disease, do not understand the information they do receive, and do not understand treatment at the time of their visit. Since providers rarely have the extensive time necessary to fully educate their patients and patients do not have the time to develop questions, providers should encourage patients to join the National Psoriasis Foundation.

The National Psoriasis Foundation is a non-profit agency dedicated to psoriasis and psoriatic arthritis. They provide many educational resources (Table 1). They have a monthly publication titled *Advance Psoriasis*, a variety of brochures, webinars, and online articles ranging in topics, including psoriasis symptoms, types of psoriasis, treatments, related conditions, comorbidities, and living with psoriasis. The website provides a means to become involved in a community of patients with psoriasis through message boards, blogs, and social media pages. By becoming part of a community it may help combat the feelings of isolation and depression patients with psoriasis often experience. In addition, it provides information on current research efforts and opportunities to become involve with advocacy. Patients can join the National Psoriasis Foundation through their website, www.psoriasis.org.

Other resources patients may find beneficial include the International Federation of Psoriasis Associates (http://www.ifpa-pso.org/) and The Psoriasis Association (www.psoriasis-association.org.uk/). By assisting patients to find reliable resources, providers can help their patients understand their disease and ease anxiety, which may decrease comorbid conditions and increase adherence, ultimately improving treatment outcomes.

Tips and Tricks

1. Encourage the patient to become enrolled in the National Psoriasis Foundation

2. Use the patient's visit to establish good rapport, as this will ease their anxiety of treating psoriasis and can likely improve adherence

Suggested Resources:
www.psoriasis.org
www.ifpa-pso.org
www.psoriasis-association.org.uk

Table 1. Resources available through the National Psoriasis Foundation.

Psoriasis and Psoriatic Arthritis Information Kit	Overview booklet that contains information about the disease, answers common questions about treatment options, and provides tips for decreasing symptoms
	List of resources for support, insurance help, and financial assistance
	Information about National Psoriasis Foundation events
TalkPsoriasis.org	Online community that allows you to connect with other members of TalkPsoriasis.com to exchange information and meet others that are affected by psoriasis or psoriatic arthritis
	Event calendar to learn about events near you
Psoriasis Advance	Quarterly magazine publication
	Includes updates on research, individual's anecdotes, tips for healthy living, treatment, and how to become an effective advocate
E- Newsletters	Free e newsletters
	Includes information on current research, treatments, advocacy, and tips for living with psoriasis and psoriatic arthritis
	Care e-newsletters with information for providers; sent 4 times per year
	Cure e-newsletters on research, advancements, and treatments for psoriasis and psoriatic arthritis; sent 6 times per year

	Learn e-newsletters include educational information and advice on living with psoriasis and psoriatic arthritis; sent monthly *Walk* e-newsletters include opportunities to get involved in the NPF Walk to Cure Psoriasis events; sent 4 times per year
Educational Booklets	Over 15 free educational booklets available for download from their websites Topics include: About psoriasis and psoriatic arthritis, treating psoriasis and psoriatic arthritis, and family guides Printed versions also available
Webcasts	Provide up-to-date information on psoriasis and psoriatic arthritis from professionals in dermatology and rheumatology Topics range but include treatments, how to live well with psoriasis, research, and accessing care
Doctor Tell Me Blog	Questions answered by experts in dermatology, rheumatology, mental health and wellness Provides the latest information for psoriasis and psoriatic arthritis
It Works for Me Blog	Treatment tips from individuals that are affected by psoriasis and psoriatic arthritis
Frequently Asked Questions (FAQ)	FAQ page for psoriasis that includes symptoms, diagnosis, types of psoriasis, severity, and triggers FAQ page for psoriatic arthritis that includes the definition, symptoms, diagnosis and treatments
Health Educator	Able to ask questions to a health educator either via email or telephone
Physician Directory	Directory of professional members of the National Psoriasis Foundation

Table 2. Checklist for Patient Resources and Education

1.	Provide the patient with general information regarding psoriasis, treatment options, and the chronicity of the disease.	
2.	Encourage the patient to join a psoriasis group, such as the National Psoriasis Foundation.	
3.	Ask the patient if they have any other questions.	

Chapter 3: Psoriatic Arthritis and Other Comorbidities

Kathryn L. Anderson

The second step in treatment of psoriasis, after assuring the patient is familiar with reliable resources such as the National Psoriasis Foundation, is assessing the patient for joint pain and other co-morbidities (Table 1). It is recommended that comorbidities be assessed annually, if not at every visit.

Table 1. Comorbidities associated with psoriasis.

Psoriatic Arthritis
Obesity
Diabetes
Metabolic Syndrome
Hypertension
Dyslipidemia
Depression
Alcohol Abuse
Positive Smoking History
Crohn's Disease
Ulcerative Colitis
Non-Alcoholic Fatty Liver Disease
Chronic Kidney Disease
Malignancy (Non-Melanoma Skin Cancer

Psoriatic Arthritis

The prevalence of psoriatic arthritis is estimated to be between 20 and 30% of patients with psoriasis. Clinically, the symptoms of psoriatic arthritis can vary widely, from mild stiffness to severe pain and it can affect the joints, spine, or connective tissue. Signs and symptoms of psoriatic arthritis generally do not present until 5 to 10 years after the skin lesions. The severity of the skin disease does not correlate with the extent of the joint disease. The Classification Criteria for Psoriatic Arthritis (CASPAR) includes inflammatory joint, spine, or connective tissue disease with at least 3 other indicators (Table 2).

Screening for psoriatic arthritis can be done either via either screening questions or through use of a formal screening tool. Screening questions include: (1) Do you have any new joint pain, stiffness, or swelling or back pain? (2) If yes, when is the joint pain/stiffness the most severe? (3) If in the morning, how long does it take for your joints to "loosen up" or decrease in pain after you get out of bed? If the patient answers that it takes longer than 60 minutes for their joints to loosen, then psoriatic arthritis is likely. Any degree of joint pain may warrant evaluation by primary care or a rheumatologist (the dermatologist can also diagnose and manage the psoriatic arthritis if he or she feels he or she meets the standard of care of a rheumatologist. We don't). . Examples of formal screening tools include the Psoriatic Arthritis Screening and Evaluation (PASE) tool, Psoriatic Arthritis Questionnaire (PAQ), Toronto Psoriatic Arthritis Screening (ToPAS) tool, Early Arthritis for Psoriatic patients (EARP) questionnaire, and the Psoriasis Epidemiology Screening ProjecT (PEST).

In addition, during the physical exam at a dermatology visit, the joints in the hands and feet can be assessed for swelling and structural irregularities, which also may suggest psoriatic arthritis, and warrant a referral to rheumatology for further workup. In addition, if patients have nail changes— such as pitting, onycholysis, or oil spots— they are at an increased risk of also having psoriatic arthritis.

The most important aspect when screening for psoriatic arthritis is to use a highly sensitive method and refer to a rheumatologist for a definitive diagnosis and treatment plan, as the disease has the potential to progress and cause debilitating joint destruction.

Table 2. Classification Criteria for Psoriatic Arthritis (CASPAR)

Inflammatory joint, spine, or connective tissue disease with at least 3 of the following:
Personal history of psoriasis (counts as 2)
Family history of psoriasis
Psoriatic nail changes (including pitting, oil drops or salmon patches, onycholysis, and Beau lines)
Negative test for rheumatoid factor
History of dactylitis
Radiologic evidence of juxtaarticular bone formation

Cardiovascular Comorbidities

Psoriasis is potentially associated with multiple cardiovascular (CV) risk factors, including obesity (prevalence in psoriasis: 8-73%, odds ratio: 1.39-1.49), diabetes (7-41%, 1.20-2.80), metabolic syndrome (16-40%, 1.30-5.92), hypertension (13-50%, 1.09-3.27), and dyslipidemia (6-61%, 1.00-2.09). Not surprisingly, with increased prevalence of CV risk factors and potentially due to the chronic inflammation of psoriasis, there is an increased risk of major CV events including myocardial infarction (relative risk (RR): 1.70, 95% confidence interval (CI): 1.11-1.74), stroke (RR: 1.56, 95% CI: 1.32-1.84), and CV mortality (RR: 1.39, 95% CI: 1.11-1.74).

It is recommended that patients with psoriasis receive age-appropriate screening of blood pressure, body mass index, waist circumference, lipids profile, fasting glucose, glycosylated hemoglobin, and smoking status at the time of diagnosis and annually thereafter. This screening can be done by dermatology, cardiology, endocrinology, or primary care. If any of the screening tests are abnormal the patient should be monitored and managed appropriately, most commonly by primary care, cardiology, and/or endocrinology.

Since obesity is associated with more severe psoriasis, it may be beneficial to discuss weight loss, dietary modifications, and lifestyle changes at dermatology visits.

Psychological Comorbidities

A variety of psychological conditions are associated with psoriasis, possibly because a decrease in their ability to work, time consumption of treatments, stigmatization, or other consequences of psoriasis that can lead to a decrease in quality of life. The prevalence of depression in patients with psoriasis is estimated to be 15-62%, compared to 6.2% in the United States adult population. The prevalence of alcohol abuse and smoking is increased in patients with psoriasis, 15-30% and 30-51% respectively, with hazard ratios of 1.39-1.49 and 3.10-3.61.

It is important to screen for these psychological conditions in patients with psoriasis, not only to identify their presence, but these untreated psychological conditions can lead to inadequate treatment of psoriasis due to decrease adherence or inappropriate treatment.

Like psoriatic arthritis, screening for these conditions can be done via informal screening questions or by formal questionnaires. Examples of questionnaires that can be used include the Patient Health Questionnaire (PHQ-9) for depression and the CAGE questionnaire for alcohol abuse.

The results of these screening measures or responses to questions during the patient interview may influence your treatment recommendations. If there is suspicion that a patient has depression, referral to a psychiatrist for formal evaluation and management may be warranted.

Inflammatory Bowel Disease

Psoriasis is associated with both Crohn's disease and ulcerative colitis, and there is an even higher prevalence of these inflammatory bowel diseases in patients with psoriatic arthritis. Many of the systemic medications used to treat psoriasis, including methotrexate and the TNF-alpha inhibitors, can also be used to treat inflammatory bowel disease.

The review of systems can include questions about gastrointestinal symptoms; including stomach pains, diarrhea, constipation, blood in the stools, or bowel urgency. However, it should be kept in mind that many medications used to treat psoriasis can also be associated with gastrointestinal side effects. If the patient has any of the above symptoms and they are not likely a medication side effect, a referral to their primary care provider or a gastroenterologist for further work-up may be necessary.

Other Comorbidities

Other comorbidities may be associated with psoriasis. These include non-alcoholic fatty liver disease, chronic kidney disease, and malignancies, specifically non-melanoma skin cancer. More research is needed to determine the associations.

Tips and Tricks

1. Be familiar with the comorbidities associated with psoriasis (Figure 1).

2. Assess the patient yearly for signs and symptoms of psoriatic arthritis.

3. Use the review of systems during the patient interview to assess for possible comorbidities.

4. Refer patients to a primary care provider, cardiologist, endocrinologist, gastroenterologist, or psychiatrist when appropriate.

Suggested References:

1) Strohal R, Kirby B, Puig L. Psoriasis beyond the skin: an expert group consensus on the management of psoriatic arthritis and common co-morbidities in patients with moderate-to-severe psoriasis. *J Eur Acad Dermatol Venereol* 2013.

2) Gottlieb AB, Dann F. Comorbidities in patients with psoriasis. *Am J Med* 2009;122(12):1150-1159.

Table 3. Checklist for Assessing for Comorbidities

1.		Assess the patient for signs and symptoms of psoriatic arthritis through a questionnaire, the patient interview, and/or the physical exam.	
	A.	Assess for symptoms and risk factors for psoriatic arthritis Pain, swelling, or morning stiffness in joints or back?	
		Neck, back, or hip tenderness?	
		Family history of psoriasis?	
		Swelling of fingers or toes?	
	B.	Assess for signs of psoriatic arthritis Nails: pitting, onycholysis, hyperkeratosis	
		Fingers and Toes: swelling/dactylitis	
		Hands: warm and/or tender joints	
		Feet: Achilles tendonitis or plantar fasciitis	
	C.	If any of the above are positive, refer patient to rheumatology for definitive diagnosis and treatment plan	
2.		Assess the patient for cardiovascular comorbidities.	
	A.	Order and/or review:	
		Cardiovascular personal and family history (myocardial infarctions, strokes, CV death)	
		Blood Pressure (>140/90 on two consecutive measurements)	
		Body Mass Index (BMI > 30 kg/m^2)	
		Waist Circumference (>88cm in woman and >102cm in men)	
		Lipid Profile (TC $\geq$ 240 mg/dL; LDL $\geq$ 130 mg/dL; HDL $\leq$ 40 mg/dL; TG $\geq$ 200 mg/dL)	
		Fasting Glucose ($\geq$126 mg/dL)	
		Glycosylated Hemoglobin (> 6.5%)	
		Smoking Status	
	B.	If any of the above are abnormal, discuss with the patient who they would like to follow-up with, and make the appropriate referral (usually to primary care, cardiology, or endocrinology)	
	C.	Discuss weight loss, dietary changes, and lifestyle modifications and how they can impact psoriasis.	
3.		Assess the patient for psychiatric comorbidities	

A.	Asses the patient for depression, either with a questionnaire or the patient interview Does the patient feel down, depressed, or hopeless?	
	Do they have little interest or pleasure in doing things?	
B.	Refer to psychiatry if depression is suspected	
C.	Assess alcohol abuse, either with a questionnaire or the patient interview	
D.	Assess smoking status	
E.	Modify treatment recommendations as necessary	
4.	Assess the patient for symptoms of inflammatory bowel disease	
A.	Does the patient have stomach pains, diarrhea, blood in their stool, or bowel urgency?	
B.	If yes to part 4A, complete a referral to the patient's primary care provider or a gastroenterologist.	
5.	Assess for other potential comorbidities	
A.	Does the patient have any signs of malignancy such as unintentional weight loss, night sweats, swollen and painless lymph nodes?	
B.	Does the patient have signs of nonalcoholic fatty liver disease? Does the patient have an AST, ALT, and/or GGT elevated twice the upper limit of normal in 2 consecutive tests with the presence of other risk factors (history of diabetes mellitus, hypertension, obesity, metabolic syndrome, or dyslipidemia)	
C.	If yes to 5A and/or 5B complete a referral to the patient's primary care provider	

Chapter 4: Adherence and the Treatment of Psoriasis

Kathryn L. Anderson

Introduction

Adherence is the degree to which a patient follows the treatment regimen agreed upon between the patient and the physician. Non-adherence is a prevalent problem in all specialties of medicine, and creates a barrier for successful treatment of many conditions. Treatment for chronic conditions, like psoriasis, carry a larger non-adherence burden.

Adherence can be divided into primary adherence, obtaining and starting the recommended treatment, and secondary adherence, maintaining treatment. In dermatology, primary non-adherence is about 30% across all conditions, however when limited to psoriasis, *primary non-adherence is about 50%*, the worst of all dermatologic conditions studied. Secondary adherence is also poor in the treatment of psoriasis with a rate between 22-67%, including discontinuing treatment, using the incorrect dosage, or using incorrect frequency.

Reasons for poor adherence

Many issues have been cited as reasons for non-adherence in the treatment of psoriasis (Table 1). Some studies have suggested that sociodemographic factors such as age, gender, and marital status affect adherence with women, teenagers, and single individuals being less compliant, although this is not consistent across all studies. Financial status may also play a role, as some patients may have difficulty affording treatment. Severity of disease impacts adherence, with patients with more severe disease usually being *less* adherent to their therapy. Type of treatment is related to adherence. Systemic treatments tend to have better adherence than topical treatments, and there is variability within each of these larger divisions based on class of systemic or vehicle of topical. The messy and time consuming nature of applying topical medications may contribute to its lower adherence compared to systemic medications. The potential and/or experienced side effects of the medications can lead to poor adherence. Patients with a poor quality of life tend to be less adherent to their medication regimen, as well as patients who are psychologically distressed, including patients suffering from depression.

If a patient is not satisfied with their treatment they are less likely to be adherent. Many aspects will affect a patient's satisfaction with treatment including efficacy, cosmetic effects, messiness, and frequency of use. Lastly, adherence is affected by the patient's satisfaction with their provider and the patient-provider trust. Poor adherence to treatment is a complex issue, and it is likely that multiple factors play a role depending on the individual patient.

Table 1. Reasons for non-adherence in the treatment of psoriasis.

Sociodemographic Factors (age, gender, social stigma, employment, financial status, marital status)
Severity of Disease
Type of Treatment Prescribed
Lifestyle Factors
Patient's Quality of Life
Psychological Distress
Patient's Satisfaction with Treatment
Patient's Satisfaction with Patient- Provider Relationship

Adherence to Topical Therapies

Patients with mild-to-moderate psoriasis— often defined as less than 10% of body surface area affected (BSA) but more practically defined as few enough spots that topicals can be realistically applied to all the lesions— are generally managed with topical treatments. Regardless of the definition, if a provider and/or patient does not feel all lesions can be adequately treated with a topical medication due to distribution, inconvenience or other reason, then phototherapy or a systemic treatment would be appropriate.

When a topical medication is prescribed, vehicle is an important factor to consider. Standard teaching has been ointment vehicles are the most potent and effective for psoriasis. However, many patients find ointments greasy and messy. If the patient dislikes ointments and chooses to not use it, it will not be effective. Therefore it is best to discuss with the patient their vehicle preference. One vehicle is clearly better than all the others: the one the patient wants to use. Due to the minimal side effect profile and high efficacy of topical treatments when used correctly, it is ideal to maximize adherence to topical therapy before switching to a systemic therapy.

Adherence to Systemic Therapies

Adherence to phototherapy and systemic therapies for psoriasis is variable. In general, adherence to systemic treatment is better than with topicals, but overall adherence is still poor. Adherence is also generally worse with self-administered treatments than with office-administered treatments.

When adherence to the oral medication, acitretin, was compared to the adherence of home phototherapy, adherence to home phototherapy was higher, with adherence rates of 54.4% and 81% respectively. Adherence to injectable biologic medications is poor, with an average of 67% in one study. The adherence rate for ustekinumab was about 80-100% when it was administered in the office setting, suggesting that some patients on biologic medications may benefit from office-administered injections.

Means to Improve Adherence

A variety of techniques can be employed to increase adherence in the treatment of psoriasis. Adherence is higher around the time of an office visit. This phenomenon, also known as "white coat compliance," is similar to how dental flossing increases before and after a dentist visit and can be exploited in clinical practice to increase adherence. One way this can be done is through an early follow-up visit after the treatment is first prescribed. The return visit will encourage the patient to obtain and start the treatment immediately, and likely the patient will realize its benefit and continue the treatment, potentially getting in the habit of using the medication. This situation can be compared to a patient who is given a prescription and scheduled to follow-up in 8 to 12 weeks. They are less likely to receive the medication in a timely manner and use it consistently enough to see a benefit. In a different context, this is like a piano teacher who provides a student sheet music, instructs them to practice daily, and holds a recital in 8 to 12 weeks. Likely, the recital would be less impressive than a student that had weekly lessons thereby encouraging regular practice. Since a weekly follow-up is not feasible for most provider and patients, a telephone call, email, or survey system (like the one provided by Causa Research, http://www.causaresearch.com/) may provide similar benefits.

Comorbid conditions can be associated with poor adherence. Depression can lead to poor adherence due to forgetfulness or hopelessness regarding their disease. If depression is suspected, the patient can be referred to a psychiatrist for a formal evaluation and treatment. Smoking and alcohol abuse can have a negative impact on adherence. At clinic visits, these issues should be addressed and the patient should be encouraged to abstain from these habits.

Simplifying the medication regimen may also improve adherence. Combination products can be used when available, as opposed to prescribing multiple therapies which can overwhelm patients. If possible, requiring that a medication only be taken or applied once a day can have better adherence rates than a medication that requires multiple treatments per day; dosing schedules of more than twice daily are associated with particularly poor adherence.

Another way to improve adherence is to enlist help from the patient's significant other, family member, or other individual involved in their health care. This is especially helpful applying topical medications to the scalp or hard to reach locations, such as the upper back, since it will make the application of the product easier for the patient and also provide another person to remind the patient.

It is important to consider what vehicle the patient prefers, as the patient will be more apt to use the medication if they don't mind putting it on and do not find the medication messy and time consuming.

Encouraging medication adherence can lead to an overall decreased cost in the treatment of psoriasis by decreasing the need for additional office visits and medication changes. The resulting better options can also decrease patient's frustration with their treatment. However, adherence is a complex issue with multiple factors affecting it and developing a single solution that works for all patients is difficult.

Tips and Tricks

1. Schedule an early follow-up with the patient. Asking the patient to call, email, or complete a survey to report how their medication is working one week after the initial visit can be used instead of an office visit.

2. Enlist the help of the patient's significant other or family member involved in their health care to help the patient apply topical treatments, especially when treating scalp psoriasis.

3. Consider patients' preferences when making treatment decisions, particularly in terms of vehicle for topical treatment.

4. Assess for comorbidities (smoking status, alcohol consumption, depression) that may be related to poor adherence.

Suggested References

1) Levender MM, Fledman SR. Adherence to drug therapy. In: Wolverton SE, editor. *Comprehensive Dermatologic Drug Therapy*. 3rd ed. Elsevier; 2013.

2) Thorneloe RJ, Bundy C, Griffiths CE, Ashcroft DM, Cordingley L. Adherence to medication in patients with psoriasis: a systematic literature review. *Br J Dermatol* 2013;168(1):20-31.

3) Chan SA, Hussain F, Lawson LG, Ormerod AD. Factors affecting adherence to treatment of psoriasis: comparing biologic therapy to other modalities. *J Dermatolog Treat* 2013;24(1):64-69.

4) Causa Research: A simple solution for a complex problem. 2014. 10-20-2014. Ref Type: Online Source (www.causaresearch.com)

Table 2. Checklist of measures that can be used to improve adherence

1.		General Measures to Improve Adherence	
	A.	Build patient-provider trust	
		Educate patient on their disease (can enlist the help of nurses and recommend the patient become a member of the National Psoriasis Foundation)	
		Acknowledge the burden of their disease	
		Touch their psoriasis lesions during physical exam	
	B.	Schedule an early follow-up with the patient (an appointment, telephone call, email, online survey (such as the one provided through Causa Research), or other means of communication)	
	C.	Assess and address comorbidities	
		Screen for depression and refer to psychiatry when appropriate	
		Assess for alcohol abuse and discuss options to receive help	
		Assess smoking status and discuss the importance of quitting and options for help	
	D.	Assess the treatment regimen to determine if it is as simplified as possible	
		Minimal frequency of medication use/application (ideally no more than once a day)	
		Minimal number of products	
		Combination products when appropriate	
2.		Measures to Improve Adherence to Topical Therapies	
	A.	Demonstrate the proper way to apply topical medications	
	B.	Determine if the patient is willing to apply topical treatment to all lesions	
	C.	Determine which vehicle the patient prefers	

Chapter 5: Treatment of localized (mild-to-moderate) psoriasis

Michael E. Farhangian

Introduction

Topical medications are used to treat psoriasis in patients with "mild-to-moderate" psoriasis, basically in patients who are willing and able to regularly apply medication to their spots. Since 80% of people with psoriasis suffer from limited psoriasis (and since topicals are also prescribed to treat the more resistant spots in patients on phototherapy or systemic treatments), topical treatment is a quintessential aspect of managing the psoriasis in the vast majority of patients. The main topical treatment options include high (and superhigh) potency topical corticosteroids, topical steroids used with a separate vitamin D_3 analogue, and a single combination product that contains both (Figure 1, Table 1). Sensitive areas such as the face or intertriginous areas may warrant treatment with weaker corticosteroids or calcineurin inhibitors, or, perhaps more practically, with short term use of the more potent agents that are being prescribed for other areas.

The extent and location of the patients' disease, as well as patients' personal preference and tolerability of side effects, will determine the treatment that suits them best. Patient preferences are critical to consider because adherence to topical medications is even lower than adherence to oral medications and represents the major hurdle to success with topical treatment. Patients may find applying some topical medications to be cumbersome and messy, so prescribing a medication that a patient will actually use can make all the difference.

Localized phototherapy can also be used in patients with localized psoriasis. Laser and non-laser, office and home-based, options are available. These approaches are discussed in Chapter 6.

Table 1. Approach to treating localized psoriasis

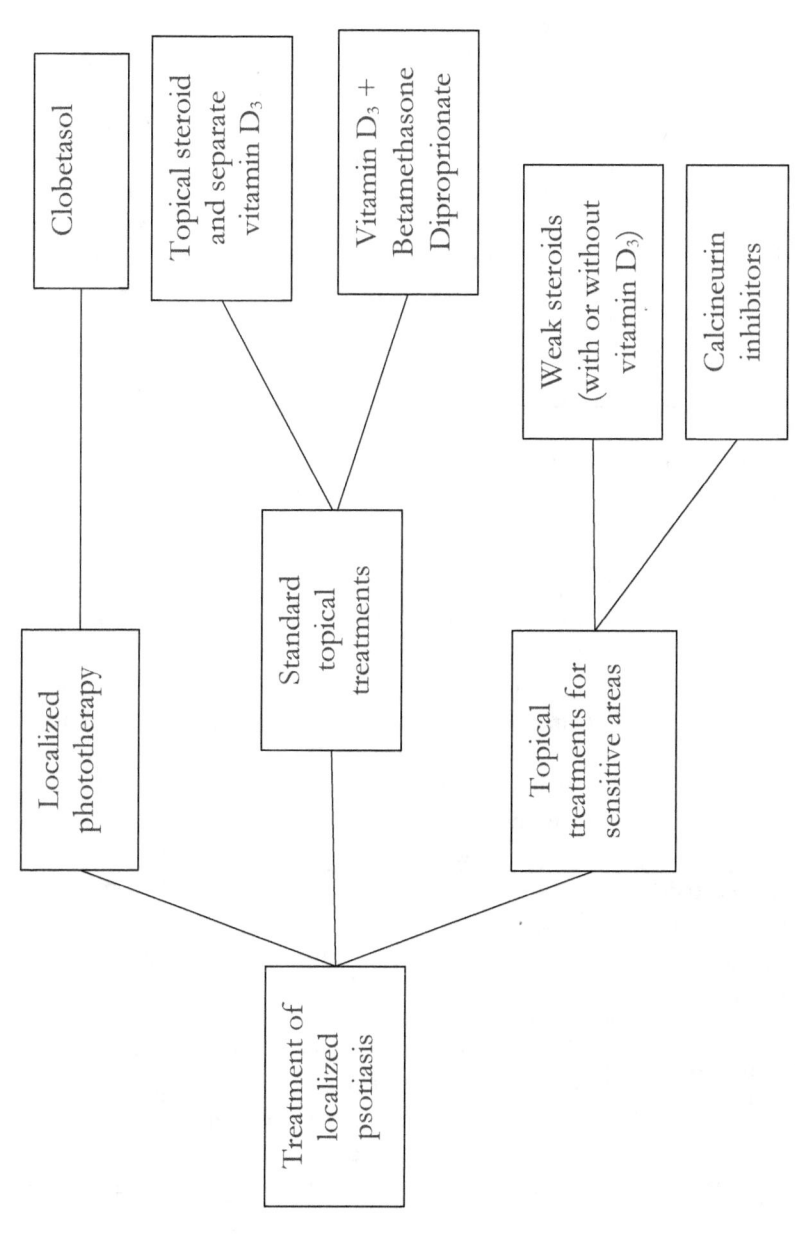

Table 1. Main Topical Treatments

Main Treatments	Background Information and Dosing	Advantages	Disadvantages
Potent Steroids (clobetasol proprionate, betamethasone diproprionate)	Approved for twice daily use for 2-4 weeks. Can be used once daily. Potent steroids are generally required for thick psoriasis plaques	Quick and effective in improving psoriatic lesions, even those that are thick and chronic Patients can see improvement in days	Increased risk of side effects with potent steroids Daily use for more than 2-4 weeks is not recommended, but patients can use them intermittently as needed for long periods
Potent Steroid + Vitamin D$_3$ (clobetasol + calcipotriene or calcitriol)	Vitamin D products work slowly and can be irritating. Use with a topical steroid speeds clearing and eliminates the irritation Calcitriol is less irritating than calcipotriene	Vitamin D use helps reduce the long term risk from potent steroid use	Expensive Prescribing multiple medications makes treatment more complicated and may reduce adherence to treatment
Potent Steroid + Vitamin D$_3$ combination medication (betamethasone diproprioinate + calcipotriene, brand name Taclonex®)	Approved as once daily, but can be used twice daily Not as potent as clobetasol, but perhaps somewhat safer.	One medication simplifies treatment regimen More effective than betamethasone diproprionate or vitamin D alone	Combination medication is expensive Side effects of potent steroids are still a risk Only available in greasy vehicles

Vehicles

Topical medications are delivered to the skin using vehicles. There are no fixed standards as to how vehicle are named, but ointments tend to be greasy, while gels, solutions and sprays tend to be far less so (Table 2). Previous dogma taught that ointments were inherently more potent, but this is no longer (if it ever was) true, especially considering the potential for poor adherence to messy ointment vehicles. Patients' personal preference and tolerance for the vehicles used will help guide which vehicle to prescribe. For instance, some patients may prefer a gel, while others may prefer a cream, a spray or even an ointment. Patients with scalp psoriasis would likely find solutions or foams to be much easier to apply than other vehicles. Cultural preference can also help choose a vehicle, as some people in some cultures may oil their scalps and prefer greasier vehicles. Providing patients with the vehicle that they prefer best can have a huge impact on their adherence to the medication.

Side Effects/Monitoring

Very rarely, patients treated with potent topical steroids and vitamin D_3 can experience systemic side effects (Table 3). Patients who are using large quantities of these medications are at increased risk. To avoid adrenal suppression from topical clobetasol, no more than 50 grams of clobetasol or 45 grams of betamethasone diproprionate should be used in a week; continuous use of clobetasol for more than 2 to 4 weeks is also to be avoided. To avoid effects of vitamin D on serum and kidney calcium, patients should not exceed 200 grams of calcitriol or 100 grams of calcipotriene in one week. Taclonex (betamethasone diproprionate + calcipotriene) should not be used in excess of 100 grams per week. Since the use of potent topical steroids is so ubiquitous in the treatment of psoriasis, it is important to keep in mind irreversible side effects such as skin atrophy and stretch marks can occur. As patients begin to see benefits from steroid treatments, it is prudent to taper their use once good clinical response is achieved. Vitamin D_3 analogs commonly cause irritation, which can make it difficult to use on sensitive skin. Trying calcitriol instead of calcipotriene or using the vitamin D product in conjunction with a topical steroid of the appropriate strength can help alleviate some of these side effects.

Table 2. Topical Medication Vehicles

Vehicles	Pros	Cons	Ideal For
Ointments	Maintains a moisture barrier Sometimes more effective at delivering medication	Messy, can ruin clothes Difficult to remove	Thick, dry scales in patients who don't mind the greasiness
Creams	Vanishes when rubbed into skin Has some emollient properties		Patients who prefer a less messy vehicle Sensitive skin
Lotions	Cooling effect which may be soothing Easy to apply		Large area of involvement and hair bearing areas
Gels	Cooling effect which may be soothing	Irritating Drying	
Foams	Leaves minimal residue Easy to spread and apply Rapidly absorbed into skin	May sting	Scalp psoriasis Large area of involvement
Solutions	Leaves minimal residue Easy to spread and apply	Alcohol content can worsen dryness and sting	Scalp psoriasis Large area of involvement

Less Commonly Prescribed Treatments

Most often, mild to moderate psoriasis can be adequately controlled using just topical corticosteroids and/or vitamin D_3 analogs. Rarely, alternative treatment options such as tazarotene, calcineurin inhibitors, and coal tar are used.

Tazarotene

Tazarotene is a topical vitamin A analog that works by decreasing the proliferation of skin cells and aiding in their proper differentiation, as well by decreasing inflammation. Like vitamin D, vitamin A drugs avoid steroid side effects, but vitamin A topical treatment can also be irritating, even more so than vitamin D topicals. Tazarotene and corticosteroids can be used in combination, with the latter helping offset the irritating effects of tazarotene, and is more effective just treating with tazarotene alone. Topical vitamin A derivatives can, at least in theory, cause birth defects and although systemic absorption of tazarotene is very limited, patients should be informed of this risk. Avoiding use of topical tazarotene in women of child bearing potential may be prudent, since other options are available.

Topical Calcineurin Inhibitors

Tacrolimus and pimecrolimus are calcineurin inhibitors that work by decreasing the release of inflammatory molecules, which play a large role in psoriasis. Having anti-inflammatory properties like steroids but without steroid side effects, they may be best used in areas with sensitive skin such as intertriginous areas and the face.

Coal Tar

Coal tar is an over the counter remedy that has been used for many years for the treatment of psoriasis. It is often poorly tolerated by patients due to its characteristic smell and because it can stain clothing. But it works. Given how poor patients' adherence to coal tar must be, coal tar must be a potent treatment.

Anthralin

Formally a commonly used topical medication for psoriasis, the use of anthralin has decreased over the years due to its potential for irritating skin and its tendency to stain anything from clothing even to ceramic bathroom fixtures.

Salicylic Acid

Salicylic acid is believed to help psoriasis by breaking down the scale that is present in psoriasis plaques. Through this mechanism, it can be used in combination with other corticosteroids or tacrolimus to theoretically improve their penetration into the skin.

Table 3. Overview of topical medications

Topical Medications	Time for good response	Common Side Effects	Rare but Severe Side Effects
Corticosteroids	2-4 weeks (longer for lower potency)	Skin thinning, dilation of capillaries, stretch marks (bigger risk in higher potency)	Systemic: Hypothalamic-pituitary-adrenal axis suppression
Coal tar products	12 weeks	May stain clothing; inflammation of hair follicles, sensitivity to sunlight; irritation of the skin	None
Tacrolimus and Pimecrolimus	8 weeks	Temporary burning and itching	Potential lymphoma
Tazaratene	8 weeks	Irritation to psoriasis lesions; sensitivity to sunlight; rash; skin discoloration	Swelling of extremities; elevated triglyceride levels; localized bleeding
Vitamin D analog	6 weeks or sooner	Temporary irritation to psoriasis lesions on skin; sensitivity to sunlight	Systemic: Reversible serum calcium elevation
Vitamin D analog/ Betamethasone	4 weeks	Temporary irritation to psoriasis lesions on skin; sensitivity to sunlight; skin thinning, dilation of capillaries, stretch marks	Systemic: Hypothalamic-pituitary-adrenal axis suppression
Anthralin	8 weeks	Skin irritation and staining of the skin	Potential kidney damage

Tips and Tricks

1. Topical treatments can be very effective if patients adhere to the treatment. Adherence to topicals is often poor. When prescribing topicals, do what you can to promote good adherence.

2. Having the patient place generic clobetasol solution in a spray bottle may be more affordable than purchasing brand name clobetasol spray products.

3. Informing pharmacists that they may dispense a different corticosteroid product of similar strength in the same vehicle if it is cheaper for the patient.

4. Use of clobetasol as needed is very effective and is less complicated compared to use of multidrug treatment regimens. Side effects from intermittent use are unlikely in real life practice, because most patients are poorly adherent to regular use of topical treatment.

5. In patients who do not mind greasy vehicles: prescribing clobetasol ointment for overnight use and having them cover the area with plastic after application of medicine may be a potent way to achieve rapid improvement in resistant lesions.

6. Consider localized ultraviolet light treatments as an alternative treatment for localized psoriasis lesions.

Table 4. Topical Treatment Checklist

Choose a topical vehicle that the patient is willing to use	
Provide patients with information about side effects and how long to expect improvement	
Inform patients that they should not exceed weekly amounts of medications:	
200g of calcitriol, 100g of calcipotrine, 50g of clobetasol, 45g betamethsone diproprionate, or 100g of combination betamethasone diproprionate + calcipotriene (Taclonex ®)	
Inform patients that they should not exceed 2-4 weeks of continuous daily superpotent topical steroid use	
Ensure patients with psoriasis on the face, intertriginous areas, and thin skinned areas are not receiving high potency steroids for daily long term use	
Schedule follow up appointment in 2-4 weeks following the prescription of potent corticosteroids to assess for response and potential side effects (see Chapter 4 on adherence for advice on how to assure good adherence to treatment)	
Ensure that patients who are pregnant or nursing are not prescribed tazarotene	

Chapter 6: Phototherapy

Kathryn L. Anderson

Introduction

Phototherapy is a first-line treatment for moderate-to-severe psoriasis (and a second-line treatment for mild-to-moderate psoriasis not responding to topical medications), able to treat a widespread area with good efficacy and a reasonable side effect profile. This chapter will provide an overview of phototherapy including mechanism of action, types of phototherapy, side effects, contraindications, and information on home phototherapy. Brief phototherapy protocols are provided, though for detailed protocols needed to run phototherapy in your office, see Phototherapy Treatment Protocols for Psoriasis and Other Phototherapy-Responsive Dermatoses, 2nd Edition by Zanolli and Feldman.

Mechanism of action

Phototherapy is hypothesized to work by local immunosuppression, inhibition of epidermal hyperproliferation and angiogenesis, and causing apoptosis of T lymphocytes within the diseased skin.

Types of Phototherapy

There are variations in phototherapy based on the wavelength of light: narrow-band ultraviolet B (NB-UVB) (311-313 nm), broad-band ultraviolet B (BB-UVB) (280-320 nm), ultraviolet A (UVA) (320-400 nm) in PUVA treatment, and 308-nm ultraviolet B, which is a localized treatment delivered by an excimer laser (Table 1).

- *NB-UVB.* The most effective wavelength (on a per joule basis) for clearing psoriasis is 313 nm UVB light. NB-UVB was developed for a wavelength range limited to 311 to 313 nm, leading to superior results and higher rates of histopathological resolution compared to BB-UVB, without any apparent significant alteration in the long-term safety profile (acute sunburn-like reactions are more common). NB-UVB has largely replaced the classic BB-UVB phototherapy for psoriasis.

- *PUVA.* Psoralen plus ultraviolet A (PUVA) is a type phototherapy that uses a medication to make the skin more sensitive to light, usually oral 8-methoxypsoralen (8-MOP), in combination with UVA light exposure. PUVA is the most efficacious phototherapy treatment for psoriasis, particularly for palmoplantar psoriasis due to deeper penetration of UVA compared to UVB. However, due to more side effects (including increased risk of skin cancer), additional contraindications, and necessity to take a systemic medication adding complexity to the regimen, NB-UVB is typically used first.

- *Excimer Laser.* Excimer laser focuses UVB therapy at localized plaques, sparing the non-affected skin from the potential side effects of repetitive UVB exposure.

Side effects

The side effect profile for BB-UVB and NB-UVB are essentially identical. PUVA therapy has the same side effect profile as UVB phototherapy with the addition of greater risk of non-melanoma skin cancer and potential increase risk of melanoma and side effects associated with taking 8-MOP, including nausea and CNS disturbances (Table 1). The skin cancer risks are far greater in fair skin populations than in patients with darker skin.

Contraindications

Phototherapy is a good treatment option for many patients as there are few contraindications. Absolute contraindications include photosensitivity diseases, including lupus erythematosus and xeroderma pigmentosum. Relative contraindications include use of photosensitizing medications (such as doxycycline or fluoroquinolones), personal or family history of melanoma, and personal history of non-melanoma skin cancer. When using psoralen plus ultraviolet A (PUVA) for phototherapy additional absolute contraindications include lactation or history of reaction to psoralen and additional relative contraindications include pregnancy or severe cardiac, liver, or renal disease. Unlike many of the other systemic treatments for psoriasis, ultraviolet B (UVB) phototherapy can be used during pregnancy and lactation, in immunocompromised individuals, and in children (with care to assure they use proper eye and genital protection).

Phototherapy protocols

The protocols for administering NB-UVB phototherapy can be determined based on minimal erythema dose (MED), the shortest amount of NB-UVB to induce erythema at 24 hours, (Table 2) or Fitzpatrick's skin type (Table 3). Lower MED and lower Fitzpatrick's skin type indicate the need for a lower starting dose and slower increases in the dose. PUVA protocol is generally based on Fitzpatrick's skin type. There is not a general consensus on a protocol for excimer laser treatment (Table 4). NB-UVB and PUVA can also be used as maintenance treatment (Table 5).

Table 2. Procedure for determining MED using NB-UVB

Well-demarcate 6 areas within a sun-protected area of the patient's skin (such as the hip or buttocks) and label them A-F. This can be done with ink or with an adhesive template from a phototherapy unit provider (http://www.daavlin.com/physicians/products/uv-therapy-accessories/2671-2/).

Expose these areas to increasing doses of NB-UVB according to Fitzpatrick's Skin Type following the appropriate dosing schedule. The remaining areas of the patient's skin should be protected by using either a hand-held phototherapy unit do deliver localized light or by covering the patient's skin with clothing if using a full-body light treatment unit.

Areas of Skin	Skin Types I-III	Skin Types IV-VI
A	$20 \ mJ/cm^2$	$60 \ mJ/cm^2$
B	$30 \ mJ/cm^2$	$70 \ mJ/cm^2$
C	$40 \ mJ/cm^2$	$80 \ mJ/cm^2$
D	$50 \ mJ/cm^2$	$90 \ mJ/cm^2$
E	$60 \ mJ/cm^2$	$100 \ mJ/cm^2$
F	$80 \ mJ/cm^2$	$120 \ mJ/cm^2$

At 24 hours post-exposure, reexamine the patient to determine the lowest dose that caused erythema

Table 3. Fitzpatrick's Skin Type

Skin Type	Description based on history and physical exam
I	Always burns; never tans
II	Always burns; occasionally tans
III	Sometimes burns; always tans
IV	Never burns; always tans
V	Never burns; Brown
VI	Never burns; Black

Table 1: Types of light typically used for phototherapy for psoriasis.

	NB-UVB	PUVA	Excimer Laser
Description	Light treatment administered in office or with home phototherapy units; Treatment for plaque and guttate psoriasis; May not be as effective as PUVA for palmo-plantar psoriasis	Light treatments are administered approximately an hour after ingestion of an oral photosensitizing agent (8-methoxypsoralen); alternative forms use a bath or topical photosensitizer	Phototherapy is administered at a wavelength of 308nm to localized plaques minimizing widespread side effects
Efficacy	About 80% of patients clear with 3 treatments per week; More effective than BB-UVB; not as effective as PUVA but has fewer side effects	About 90% of patients clear after 30 treatments; Most effective form of phototherapy; Useful for palmo-plantar psoriasis because UVA penetrates deeper than UVB	Clearance of plaques in less than 12 treatments; remission for usually 4-6 months and up to 2 years
Side Effects	• Short-term: erythema, pruritus, subacute phototoxicity, herpes simplex recurrence • Long-term: photoaging (hyperpigmentation, hypopigmentation, wrinkling, actinic keratosis), non-melanoma skin cancers	• Short-term: nausea, erythema, pruritus, subacute phototoxicity, phytophotodermatitis, herpes simplex recurrence, CNS disturbances (headaches, insomnia, hyperactivity, mild depression) • Long-term: photoaging (hyperpigmentation, hypopigmentation, wrinkling, actinic keratosis), non-melanoma skin cancers, melanoma	Erythema, blisters, epidermal erosions, hyperpigmentation

Table 4. Protocols for clearing psoriasis with NB-UVB, PUVA, and excimer laser.

	Frequency	Based on MED:	Based on Fitzpatrick's Skin Type:		Managing Treatment:
			Initial Dose (mJ/cm²):	Incremental Increases (mJ/cm²):	
NB-UVB	3-4 times per week	• Initial dose: 50% MED • Treatments 1-20: increase by 10% of the MED • Treatments > 20: ordered by physician	I: 300 mJ/cm² II: 300 mJ/cm² III: 500 mJ/cm² IV: 800 mJ/cm² V: 800 mJ/cm² VI: 800 mJ/cm²	I: 100 mJ/cm² II: 100 mJ/cm² III: 125 mJ/cm² IV: 125 mJ/cm² V: 150 mJ/cm² VI: 150 mJ/cm²	• Instruct the patient to apply an emollient, such as mineral oil, prior to treatment; wear eye protection; and men a genital shield • If the patient is receiving therapy 3-4 times per week, increase the dose according to schedule* • If there has been 4-7 days since last treatment keep the dose the same; if it has been 1-2 weeks decrease dose by 25%; if it has been 2-4 weeks decrease dose by 50%; if longer than 4 weeks go back to initial dose • Do not exceed 4x the MED or 2000mJ/cm² for skin types I and II, 3000 mJ/cm² for III and IV, or 5000 mJ/cm² for V and VI

PUVA	2-3 times per week	I: 1 J/cm^2 II: 1 J/cm^2 III: 2 J/cm^2 IV: 2 J/cm^2 V: 4 J/cm^2 VI: 4 J/cm^2	I: 0.5 J/cm^2 II: 1.0 J/cm^2 III: 1.0 J/cm^2 IV: 1.0 J/cm^2 V: 1.0 J/cm^2 VI: 1.0 J/cm^2	• Instruct patients to avoid additional UV exposure for the rest of the day and use SPF 15 sunscreen on sun exposed skin • Instruct the patient to take the 8-MOP (often Oxsoralen Ultra, prescribed at 0.5-0.6 mg/kg) 1 hour prior to their treatment. Treatment needs to be given between 1 hour and 15 minutes and 1 hour and 45 minutes following the 8-MOP • Instruct all patients to wear eye protection and men to wear a genital shield • If the patient is receiving therapy 2-3 times per week, increase the dose according to schedule* • If there has been 4-7 days since last treatment keep the dose the same; if it has been 1-2 weeks decrease dose by 25%; if it has been 2-3 weeks decrease dose by 50%; if it has been 3-4 weeks

		decease the dose by 50%; if longer than 4 weeks go back to initial dose
Excimer Laser		• There are no consensus guidelines for the use of UVB Excimer Laser • Clinical studies have used initial doses ranging from 0.5MED to 16MED with some studies using a fixed dose and others increasing the dose up to 30% with each treatment • Other studies have based doses on the induration of the plaque, increasing the dose until the thickness starts to improve, then decreasing the dose as the plaque improves • Higher doses result in more rapid improvement and longer remissions but are associated with more adverse reactions, including blistering and erythema

* If the patient has remaining skin pinkness or had erythema that resolved after the last treatment, keep the dose the same. If the patient has symptomatic erythema of the skin, skip the treatment and decrease the dose by 25% at the next treatment.

Table 5. Protocols for maintenance phototherapy for psoriasis.

	Protocol for maintenance therapy
NB-UVB	(If psoriasis has cleared > 75%) • Once a week at the last dose of clearance phototherapy for 4 weeks • Decrease the dose by 25% and administer phototherapy once every 2 weeks for long-term maintenance
PUVA	(If psoriasis has cleared > 75%) • Once a week treatment at the last dose of clearance phototherapy for 4 weeks • Decrease the dose by 25% and administer phototherapy once every 2 weeks for long-term maintenance • Option to decrease the dose again by 25% and administer phototherapy once every 2-4 weeks

Other Options in Phototherapy

Home Phototherapy

Home light units are an alternative means of administering phototherapy as opposed to office-based phototherapy. Home units may be more convenient and may decrease the financial burden of office-based phototherapy due to high cost from copays, lost wages, and cost of travel for some patients. Home phototherapy can be as efficacious as office-based phototherapy with potentially greater patient satisfaction with treatment.

There are multiple companies that supply a variety of home phototherapy units (Table 6). The type of unit prescribed will depend on the patient (Table 7). The process of obtaining the unit differs depending on the company, but in general consists of the provider completing a prescription and a letter of medical necessity and the patient completing an insurance form, order form, and sales agreement. After the necessary paperwork is submitted, the company supplying the home phototherapy unit processes the insurance claim and assists the patient in obtaining the unit (Table 6 and 10). The majority of patients receive some assistance from their insurance company for coverage for the home phototherapy unit. If the patient is initially denied coverage, a smaller, less expensive unit may be tried (such as trying a multi-directional unit instead of a cabinet unit) or the patient can work with the phototherapy company to establish a payment plan.

Like patients undergoing office-based phototherapy, patients receiving a home phototherapy unit also need a treatment schedule (Table 8). Treatments are usually prescribed based on Fitzpatrick skin type and are performed every other day or 3 to 5 times per week. After 15-20 treatments most patients see at 50% improvement. Treatment should continue until the patient is clear, stops seeing improvement, or there is an adverse event. The patient should be informed that if symptomatic erythema is experienced the treatment should be held until it resolves and then re-initiated at 50% of the dose that caused the erythema. As with office-based phototherapy, the patients need to be informed about the importance of wearing eye shields and men need to be informed of the importance of genital shields.

Table 6. Companies that provide home phototherapy units.

Company	Brief Description of their Units	Offer help with insurance claims?
National Biological Corporation	Full-body cabinet, flat panels of multiple sizes, tri-fold unit, portable spot treatment units, hand/foot units; NB-UVB, BB-UVB, UVA	Yes
Daavlin	Full-body cabinet, flat panels of multiple sizes, tri-fold unit, portable spot treatment units, hand/foot units; NB-UVB, BB-UVB, UVA	Yes
UVBioTek	Full-body cabinet, tri-fold unit, flat panel unit, portable flat panel unit; NB-UVB, BB-UVB	Yes
SolarC	Single panels that can be combined to form a multidirectional unit, single panel units, table top panel, portable spot treatment unit; NB-UVB, BB-UVB	No

Tanning Beds

Commercial tanning beds are an efficacious treatment for psoriasis and have a role for in treatment. The treatment schedule can be based on Fitzpatrick's skin type, and has limitations as it has only been defined for skin types I-III, were based on recommendations from the manufacturer in the study (Wolff Technology), and the frequency of treatments per week was not standardized (Table 9); additionally, since the output of tanning beds at different establishments may vary wildly, starting slowly and increasing as tolerated may be prudent.

As with all treatments, tanning beds carry side effects; side effects include erythema, pruritus, and increased risk of melanoma and non-melanoma skin cancers. The risks must be weighed against the benefits, just as in any other treatment, and for some patients tanning beds may be the best treatment option, particularly if patients have moderate-to-severe psoriasis, have contraindications to systemic medications, and are unable to have in-office or home phototherapy due to prohibitive cost or distance from the phototherapy site. The efficacy of tanning beds can be increased with concomitant use of acitretin. However, ***oral psoralen and tanning beds should be avoided as this combination may be associated with fatal burns***.

A skin exam can be performed at 6 weeks to assess for improvement with commercial tanning bed treatment. The patient should be instructed to perform self-skin exams and have a skin exam by a dermatologist regularly to assess for side effects such as melanoma and non-melanoma skin cancers. As with other forms of phototherapy the patient should be informed of the importance of eye shields and genital shields for men.

Table 7. Variety of units available for home phototherapy.

Type of Unit	Description
Cabinet unit	Usually four panels that emit light allowing the whole body surface area to be treated with one treatment per day; ideal for patients with a large body surface area affected by psoriasis; most expensive style unit
Multi-directional unit	Typically three panels that emit light allowing multiple body surface areas to receive treatment with one treatment per day; ideal for patients with a large body surface area; if the patinet's front and back are affected they will require two treatments per day; often a good compromise between cost and time for treatment
Panel Units	Usually 6' in height but a few 4' panels available; able to treat one surface area of the body at a time; may have to do multiple treatments per day if the patient has multiple surface areas affected
Small Panels	Compact panel units ideal for spot treatment or for treatment of hands and feet; may also be a good option for patient's that need a panel unit that is portable; may be incorporated into a unit designed for hand and feet treatment
Handheld Units	Ideal for spot treatment or for scalp treatment; small, compact units that are portable; often come with a brush-like attachment for treatment of the scalp

Table 8. Example of a treatment schedule for home phototherapy with NB-UVB based on Fitzpatrick skin type.

Fitzpatrick Skin type	Initial Treatment Dose (mJ/cm²)	Increase Increments (mJ/cm²)
I	130	15
II	220	25
III	260	40
IV	330	45
V	350	60
VI	400	65

Table 9. Example of a phototherapy schedule for a commercial tanning bed.

	Treatment Time (in min)					
Skin Type	Week 1	Week 2	Week 3	Week 4	Week 5	Week 6
I	2	4	10	15	20	25
II and III	3	7	15	20	25	30

Combination Therapy

Topicals with Phototherapy

The classic phototherapy treatments, Goekermann treatment and Ingram regimen, use a combination of UVB phototherapy with topical coal tar and topical anthralin, respectively. Both treatments are highly effective but not often used clinically due to the time-consuming and messy nature of the treatments.

Emollients, such as mineral oil or petrolatum, are topical agents that can be used with phototherapy in order to facilitate the transmission of UV radiation.

Corticosteroids with UVB phototherapy, although commonly used, does not increase the efficacy over UVB phototherapy alone. In the phototherapy setting, topical corticosteroids may be most helpful for lichenified lesions that have secondary lichen simplex chronicus.

The use of vitamin D analogues in combination with UVB phototherapy can be helpful. Using vitamin D analogues *after* phototherapy treatments may provide a UV sparing effect without increasing adverse events, and therefore is a reasonable combination treatment to try. Application before phototherapy is not recommended, as vitamin D analogs can be inactivated by UV light. Adding a vitamin D analogue to a PUVA regimen improves the response to therapy and reduces the required cumulative UVA dose.

Tazarotene, a vitamin A analogue, with UVB phototherapy improves the efficacy over phototherapy alone, but increases the susceptibility of burning. Anecdotally, concomitant use of tazarotene with PUVA has a synergistic effect.

Phototherapy with Phototherapy Combination

Combinations of different types of phototherapy have not been widely studied. Combination of NB-UVB with PUVA may lead to faster clearing, although there may be a risk of increased photocarcinogenicity.

Phototherapy and Other Systemic Therapies

For information regarding the use of phototherapy with oral medications and biologic medications, see their respective chapters.

Tips and Tricks

1. Ensure that patients ALWAYS use eye protection during any light treatment, including UVB, UVA, and hand-held devices in-office, at home, or in commercial tanning beds. Patients receiving a photosensitizing agent need to continue to wear eye protection when in the sun for at least 24 hours following ingestion of the medication.

2. Men need to wear a genital shield, such as an athletic support.

3. UVB phototherapy is a great treatment for to consider for pregnant women, lactating women, and immunosuppressed individuals because it is generally considered safe to use in these patients, in contrast to the majority of the other systemic therapies.

4. Advise patients to use topical emollients, like mineral oil, before phototherapy as they increase UV penetration.

5. Home phototherapy is an alternative to in-office phototherapy, especially for patients who live far from the phototherapy clinic, cannot miss work, or cannot afford the phototherapy visit copays.

6. Take advantage of the assistance home phototherapy companies offer to make prescribing a home light unit easier for both you and the patient.

7. If practical sunlight is also a useful form of phototherapy. A tanning bed offers a more controlled way to get UV, however. If a patient desires phototherapy but is not able to attend office-based phototherapy and cannot afford a home unit, commercial tanning bed UV treatments can be recommended (despite the objections of some dermatologists).

Table 10. Checklist for Prescribing Phototherapy

Determine if the patient is a candidate for phototherapy (moderate-to-severe psoriasis or failed topical treatment)	
Review absolute contraindications; including photosensitizing disorder (lupus erythematosus and xeroderma pigmentosum) and, for PUVA only, lactation or history of a reaction to psoralen)	
Review relative contraindications for phototherapy; including use of phototsenzitizing medications, personal or family history of melanoma, personal history of non-melanoma skin cancer; and for PUVA pregnancy or severe cardiac, liver, or renal disease	
Provide patient with information about the protocol for phototherapy and expected efficacy	
Determine what phototherapy is going to be used (most commonly NB-UVB)	
Explain to the patient the importance of wearing eye shields and, in men, the importance of a genital shield	
Inform the patient to let the provider know if they have any changes in medication	
Schedule follow-up visits, usually every 3 months	
Schedule annual ophthalmology exams (biannually if on PUVA treatment)	
If prescribing office-based phototherapy:	
Inform the patient of the risks and benefits of office-based phototherapy	
Determine the patient's treatment schedule; including treatments per week (often 3), starting dose, and incremental increase, either based on MED or Fitzpatrick's Skin Type (Table 4)	
If prescribing PUVA, provide the patient with the prescription for 8-MOP (often Oxsoralen Ultra, prescribed at 0.5-0.6 mg/kg)	
If prescribing home phototherapy:	
Inform the patient of the risks and benefits of home phototherapy	
Enlist the assistance of a representative from one of the home phototherapy unit comanies	
Determine the type of unit to prescribe (cabinet unit, multidimensional unit, panel unit (tall or short), small panel unit, target unit) (Table 7)	
Determine the patient's treatment schedule; including treatments per week, initial dose, and suggested increase increments based on Fitzpatrick Skin Type (Table 8)	

Complete a prescription or order form depending on the company (with the type of unit, type of light, and dosing regimen)	
Compose a Letter of Medical Necessity (many companies provide examples) and may need pages from the patient's chart indicating past treatments	
Direct the patient to complete their portion of the paperwork (varies by the company but usually includes an order form, a sales agreement, HIPPA form, and enlarged copy of their insurance card)	
Direct the patient to submit the paperwork to the company (the company will then submit the claim to the patient's insurance company and will be in touch with the patient)	
The company will be in touch with the patient regarding the remainder of the process	
If suggesting commercial tanning beds:	
Inform the patient of the risk and benefits of using commercial tanning beds for the treatment of psoriasis	
Confirm the patient is not using psoralen	
Determine the treatment schedule; including sessions per week (usually 6-7) and initial dose and increase, based on Fitzpatrick's skin type (Table 9)	
Inform the patient it is best to use the same tanning bed at the same salon in order to keep their treatment consistent	
Inform the patient that if the bulbs are replaced in the tanning bed they need to be cautious due to increased strength of light and increased risk of burning	

Chapter 7: Methotrexate

Adam S. Richardson, Michael E. Farhangian, and Steven R. Feldman

Introduction

Systemic immunosuppressive medications are effective in the treatment of psoriasis by modulating the immune response, with methotrexate having been the first line treatment for many years. Although methotrexate is not as effective as biologic medications and has more severe potential side effects, insurance companies often do not cover the cost of biologics unless patients have tried and failed (or have a contraindication to) methotrexate. When no insurer is involved, skipping methotrexate and going straight to a biologic may be a good option.

Mechanism of action

Methotrexate functions through multiple mechanisms, and the entire mechanism in which methotrexate improves psoriasis is not completely understood. It used to be thought the benefits of methotrexate were a result of a decrease in the hyperproliferation of skin cells in psoriasis, however this is no longer believed to be the case. By inhibiting folate production, methotrexate down regulates T-cell activity by both inhibiting T-cell proliferation and inducing T-cell apoptosis. In addition, methotrexate increases the endogenous anti-inflammatory molecule adenosine, which may help suppress psoriasis.

Dosing

Methotrexate is typically prescribed on a weekly basis as 2.5mg pills (methotrexate solution for injection can be taken orally and is less costly than the pill form), or alternatively, it can be given intramuscularly by a healthcare professional or by patients themselves (Table 1). Administering methotrexate by intramuscular or subcutaneous injection in the office can be used to ensure adherence to treatment, as well as avoiding first pass hepatic effects (this approach can also be tried in patients who have nausea from oral delivery). Methotrexate is cleared by the kidneys, so those with mildly impaired renal function require a lower dose (methotrexate should not be used in patients with severely impaired renal function). Patients who are at risk for renal insufficiency, such as elderly and diabetics, can have their creatinine and glomerular filtration rate evaluated before starting therapy or a lower test dose (2.5mg) can be used.

Table 1. Methotrexate dosing

Initial dose:	5 mg test dose (2.5mg may be given in patients expected to have slightly impaired renal function, for example patients 70 years of age or older) The test dose should be followed with labs one week later to evaluate for hematological toxicity
Timing	Taken all at once, only once a week An alternative regimen of 3 divided doses given over 24 hours (the second dose 12 hours after the first, and the third dose 12 hours after that) used to be commonly used (for example, the weekly dose of 15 mg would be given as 5mg 3 times with 12 hours between each dose)
Dosage range	Typically 7.5 mg to 25 mg
Titration	The weekly dose can be increased in 5mg increments (2.5mg increments in patients who might have slightly impaired renal function) each week until a stable dose is achieved.

Efficacy

The efficacy of systemic treatments for psoriasis are generally measured using the Psoriasis Area and Severity Index (PASI) score, which rates the psoriasis severity on the basis of induration, scaliness and erythema as well as body surface area involvement. Higher PASI scores are suggestive of worse disease and a 75% improvement in PASI (so-called PASI75) is often used as a measure of success. PASI75 rates for methotrexate vary in different studies, with 30-60% of patients being treated with methotrexate achieving a PASI75 at 12 weeks of treatment. Methotrexate's PASI75 is less than that of PUVA and several biologics.[1] Patients generally start seeing some improvement in their psoriasis after approximately 4 weeks of treatment with methotrexate.

Side Effects

Methotrexate has both major and minor side effects associated with its usage (Table 2). Separating methotrexate into 3 doses separated by 12 hours once a week or administering methotrexate intramuscularly or subcutaneously can limit gastrointestinal side effects. By titrating to the lowest effective dose, the risk of side effects is minimized since many of these side effects demonstrate a dose dependent nature.

Myelosupression is a potentially fatal side effect of methotrexate and can generally be avoided by correct dosing and regular monitoring, but drops in blood counts can occur at any time during the course of treatment. White blood cells, red blood cells, and platelets should be monitored one week after the initial dose, one week after any increase in dose and on a regular basis thereafter to watch for signs of bone marrow suppression (Table 3). Patients who are at a higher risk for myelosupression include patients with renal impairment (as occurs in advanced age). In addition, hypoalbuminemia, excessive alcohol intake, and medication interactions can all increase the risk of myelosupression.

Methotrexate is hepatotoxic. The ability of a patient's liver to manage this toxicity is variable. Hepatotoxicity may be more common in patients using methotrexate for psoriasis compared to those using methotrexate for rheumatoid arthritis. A possible cause of the higher incidence of hepatotoxicity may be due to the higher incidences of obesity, diabetes, and alcoholism among psoriasis patients. Patients who already have some degree of liver disease, such as patients who drink alcohol excessively, and those with hyperlipidemia, hepatitis, familial liver disease, diabetes, obesity, and a history of hepatotoxic substance exposure are at increased risk of hepatotoxicity due to methotrexate.

---

[1] Feldman S.R., Factors for Choosing the Right Biologic Treatment. *The Dermatologist.* 2014; 22(9): http://www.the-dermatologist.com/content/factors-choosing-right-biologic-treatment. Accessed March 3,2015.

Pulmonary fibrosis is an uncommon side effect and should be a concern with new onset respiratory symptoms without an obvious cause.

Supplementation with folate may help minimize the gastrointestinal, myelosuppressive, and hepatotoxic side effects, with the recommended dosages ranging from 1-5mg daily. However, the ideal dose of folic acid is uncertain, and the affect folic acid supplementation has on the efficacy of methotrexate is uncertain.[2] Most commonly folate is taken daily except for the day methotrexate is administered. There are alternate regimens used by clinicians, but no clear regimen is superior.

Although supplemental folate may help to minimize certain side effects, folic acid cannot be used to reverse acute methotrexate toxicity. Leukopenia, thrombocytopenia, and anemia are all signs of toxicity, and complete blood counts (CBC's) should be carefully monitored. In addition elevations in mean corpuscular volume should be monitored as a sign of megaloblastic anemia. In the event of methotrexate toxicity, patients should be treated with folinic acid (Leucovorin) at a dose of 20mg ($10mg/m^2$) in oral or parenteral form (methotrexate blocks the conversion of folic acid to folinic acid, and therefore folinic acid must be used to reverse acute methotrexate toxicity). The initial dose should be followed with 20mg doses every 6 hours. Consulting a hematologist may be prudent in cases of methotrexate toxicity resulting in bone marrow suppression.

---

[2] Strober B.E., and Menon K.: Folate supplementation during methotrexate therapy for patients with psoriasis. J Am Acad Dermatol 2005; 53: pp. 652-659

Table 2. Side effects of methotrexate[3,4]

Most common minor side effects	Nausea
	Vomiting
	Diarrhea
	Stomatitis
	Fatigue
	Malaise
	Anorexia
	Fevers
	Chills
	Dizziness
	Photosensitivity
	Alopecia
Major side effects of most concern	Hepatotoxicity
	Myelosupression
	Pulmonary fibrosis
	Gastrointestinal bleeding and ulceration

Monitoring

It is suggested to monitor for hepatotoxicity with regular liver chemistries or with a liver biopsy in specific situations (Table 3) (see Chapter 15on special situations); alternatively, having the patient evaluated by a hepatologist may be prudent in some situations.

Contraindications

Methotrexate has a number of absolute and relative contraindications (Table 4). Since methotrexate is a teratogen and abortifacient, it should not be used in patients who are pregnant or wish to become pregnant (see Chapter 15 for treating psoriasis in pregnancy). There are no studies

---

[3] Kalb RE, Strober B, Weinstein G, Lebwohl M. Methotrexate and psoriasis: 2009 National Psoriasis Foundation Consensus Conference. J Am Acad Dermatol. 2009;60(5):824-37.

confirming the teratogenic effects that methotrexate has on a fetus when the father is on methotrexate. However, guidelines suggest that males should wait approximately 3 months after discontinuation of methotrexate before attempting to conceive, although methotrexate's inhibition of male spermatogenesis is debatable.

Drug Interactions

Methotrexate patients should have their medication history evaluated for possible interactions. Medications that inhibit methotrexate's ability to bind with serum albumin can increase serum levels of methotrexate and lead to toxicity. In addition, medications that inhibit the renal excretion of methotrexate can also lead to methotrexate toxicity. Methotrexate should be used carefully in patients on other hepatotoxic mediations (Table 5).

Table 5. Methotrexate drug interactions[4]

Medications that inhibit binding to albumin	Medications that inhibits renal excretion
Salicylates	Cyclosporine
Sulfonamides	Probenecid
Diphenylhydantoin	Salicylates
Penicillins	Sulfonamides
Minocycline	Naproxen
Chloramphenicol	Ibuprofen
Trimethoprim/Sulfamethoxazole	Indomethacin
Phenytoin	Phenylbutazone
	Ciprofloxacin
	Furosemide
	Thiazide Diuretics
Common hepatotoxic medications	
Statins	
Leflunomide	
Retinoids	
Azathioprine	
Minocycline	
Barbiturates	
Ethanol	
Phenytoin	

[4] Menter A, Korman NJ, Elmets CA, Feldman SR, Gelfand JM, Gordon KB, et al. Guidelines of care for the management of psoriasis and psoriatic arthritis: section 4. Guidelines of care for the management and treatment of psoriasis with traditional systemic agents. *J Am Acad Dermatol.* Sep 2009;61(3):451-85.

56

Tips and Tricks

1.   Methotrexate can have serious side effects. Patients should be given *in writing* the risks, benefits and alternatives. The National Psoriasis Foundation's Systemic Treatment brochure is a convenient way to do this. (http://www.psoriasis.org/about-psoriasis/treatments/systemics/methotrexate)

2.   Patients should be started on a test dose (5mg or 2.5mg in the setting of renal insufficiency) of methotrexate and be followed with labs in one week (Table 1).

3.   Effective dose of methotrexate varies patient to patient (titrate to the lowest effective dose in increments of 5mg or 2.5mg in the setting of renal insufficiency). See Table 1 for dosing.

4.   Increases in methotrexate dose should be followed with labs in one week.

5.   Methotrexate should only be taken one day a week. Patients need to be made aware of this. Too often, patients forget and think they are supposed to take pills daily (Table 1).

6.   Patients who cannot tolerate oral methotrexate due to gastrointestinal side effects can try intramuscular or subcutaneous preparations. Folic acid supplementation may reduce gastrointestinal side effects (as well as other side effects).

7.   Patients should have monitoring at regular intervals to screen for major side effects (Table 3).

8.   Trimethoprim/sulfamethoxazole (Bactrim/Septra) can interact with methotrexate, cause sudden death from pancytopenia, and should be strictly avoided in patients on methotrexate. Medications should be evaluated on every patient that is being started on methotrexate (Table 5).

Table 3. Methotrexate laboratory monitoring[5,3]

1.	**Initial testing**	
	Complete blood count	
	Liver function tests	
	Renal function tests	
	Pregnancy test in women of childbearing age	
	HIV test in at risk patients	
	Tuberculosis testing (PPD)	
2.	**Hepatotoxicity monitoring in patients with no risk factors**	
	No liver biopsy is necessary	
	Monitor LFTs monthly for the 1st 6 months and 1-3 months thereafter	
	For elevations < 2-fold upper limit of normal: repeat in 2-4 weeks For elevations > 2-fold but < 3-fold upper limit of normal: closely monitor, repeat in 2-4 weeks, and decrease dose as needed For persistent elevations in 5 of 9 AST levels during a 12-month period or if there is a decline in the serum albumin below the normal range with normal nutritional status, in a patient with well-controlled disease, a liver biopsy should be preformed	
	Consider liver biopsy after 3.5-4.0 g total cumulative dosage	
	Consider switching to another agent or discontinuing therapy after 3.5-4.0 g total cumulative dosage	
	Consider continuing to follow up according to above guidelines without biopsy	
3.	**Hepatotoxicity monitoring in patients with one or more risk factors**	
	Consider delayed baseline liver biopsy (after 2-6 months of therapy to establish medication efficacy and tolerability)	
	Repeat liver biopsies after roughly 1-1.5 g of methotrexate	

Table 4. Methotrexate contraindication checklist[5]

Absolute contraindications	
Patient is pregnant or nursing	
Patient has blood dyscrasias (anemia, leukopenia, thrombocytopenia)	
Patient is currently an alcoholic	
Patient has a history of hepatitis or chronic liver disease	
Patient has a hypersensitivity to methotrexate	
Patient is immunosuppressed	
Relative contraindications	
Patient has a personal or family history of liver impairment	
Patient has renal impairment	
Patient has an active or chronic infection	
Patient has a history of hepatotoxic chemical or drug exposure	
Patient BMI is not >30	
Patient has recently had a live vaccine administered	
Patient is a diabetic	

[5] Menter A, Korman NJ, Elmets CA, Feldman SR, Gelfand JM, Gordon KB, et al. Guidelines of care for the management of psoriasis and psoriatic arthritis: section 4. Guidelines of care for the management and treatment of psoriasis with traditional systemic agents. *J Am Acad Dermatol.* Sep 2009;61(3):451-85.

Chapter 8: Acitretin

Olabola Awosika, Michael E. Farhangian, Steven R. Feldman

Introduction

Acitretin is a second generation retinoid (a vitamin A derivative) used as an oral systemic therapy for patients with psoriasis that is too extensive and/or severe for topical treatment. Due to lack of significant immunosuppression and an ability to maintain long-term clinical response with prolonged therapy, acitretin can be a good alternative for severe psoriasis that is resistant to other forms of therapy. Acitretin is a potent teratogen, however, and should not be used in women of child-bearing potential.

Acitretin's ability to regulate keratinization makes acitretin useful for reducing scale in hyperkeratotic psoriasis and making phototherapy more effective. Localized and generalized forms of pustular psoriasis and erythrodermic psoriasis may respond well to acitretin monotherapy. Acitretin may be a good choice for patients with history of melanoma, solid tumors, lymphoproliferative malignancies, or HIV because its mechanism of action does not involve significant immunosuppression.

Mechanism of Action

Acitretin functions by modulating the differentiation and proliferation of keratinocytes in the epidermis by binding to nuclear receptors responsible for gene transcription. This process reduces hyperproliferation of the rapidly dividing keratinocytes in patients with psoriasis. This helps to reduce redness, peeling, and the overall thickness of skin lesions. Acitretin also has an inhibitory effect on inflammatory molecules that induces premature maturation of keratinocytes and neutrophil chemotaxis.

Dosing

The therapeutic dosage of acitretin monotherapy is usually between 25 mg every other day and 50 mg per day. Because adverse effects tend to be dose related, the treatment can be initiated at a low dose (10 to 25 mg per day) and then raised by 10 mg biweekly. This method should be continued until adverse effects experienced by the patient make it advisable to refrain from further increasing the dosage. Since low doses of acitretin are effective in some individuals, gradual dose escalation allows for patients to receive the minimum amount of medication necessary allowing for the best clinical response to be achieved while minimizing side effects. Once an acceptable clinical response has been observed, the dose can be gradually tapered to improve tolerance. This strategy allows for maintenance of efficacy at lower doses for a very long period.

Alternatively, starting high to achieve rapid clinical improvement and then lowering the dose to avoid side effects is another approach that may be preferred by patients who are seeking rapid relief from their psoriasis, for example in patients with pustular psoriasis.

Efficacy

Acitretin is somewhat effective when used as monotherapy. In a retrospective post hoc analysis of four randomized controlled trials (RCTs) of use in generalized pustular, plaque type, severe, and erythrodermic variants, 85% of patients had 50% improvement in Psoriasis Area and Severity Index (PASI50) and 52% achieved a PASI75 after 12 weeks. Acitretin is useful for long-term maintenance therapy for plaque psoriasis. In one long-term clinical trial, acitretin was effective for plaque psoriasis with 89% of patients achieving a PASI50 and 78.4% attained a PASI75 after 12 months.

In patients with pustular psoriasis, acitretin is a first-line therapy, inducing a rapid clinical response (clearance of lesions in 10 days) in up to 84% of patients. Acitretin induced five-fold reduction in pustules after 4 weeks in two RCTs in patients with palmoplantar pustulosis. Acitretin is also effective for treating nail psoriasis, with doses of 0.2 - 0.3mg/kg attaining a mean reduction in the Nail Psoriasis Severity Index (NAPSI) score of 41% and complete clearance in 25% of patients; acitretin can, however, cause thin, brittle nails, especially when used in high doses. In general, response to acitretin is gradual with peak efficacy usually achieved in 3 to 6 months.

Acitretin is often used in combination with phototherapy. The combination of acitretin with UVB, UVA (tanning bed), or PUVA therapy is more effective than either phototherapy or acitretin alone. The clearance rate for acitretin with UV-B therapy (Re-UVB, 75%) is greater than either acitretin (42%) or UVB (35 to 41%). In addition, combination therapy reduces the overall number of phototherapy sessions and the required dosage of acitretin. Moreover, acitretin exerts anticarcinogenic effects (including normalizing abnormal epidermal cell proliferation, inhibiting tumor cell angiogenesis, and down regulating proto-oncogenes) possibly reducing the risk of skin cancer compared to monotherapy with UVB, UVA, or PUVA.

When used in combination with phototherapy, it is sometimes recommended to administer acitretin at a low dose for 2 weeks before starting phototherapy; the concern is that the photosensitizing effect of acitretin will kick in when patients are getting a high UV dose resulting in a burn. Alternatively, both acitretin and UV can be started together, with the UV dose increased only very slowly. However, for patients already on phototherapy, 25mg/day of acitretin may be prescribed while concomitantly decreasing the dosage of phototherapy by 30 to 50% in the first week to prevent phtotoxicity/burning.

The combination of calcipotriol ointment and acitretin has additive benefits on the clearance success rate. In one study, the 'clear' or 'almost clear' success rate with acitretin increased from 41% to 67% with the addition of calcipotriol. In a 12 week study, the complete clearance rate increased from 15% with acitretin alone to 40% with the addition of calcipotriol.

Caution has been advised concerning the use of methotrexate with acitretin, however the combination has been used safely in some patients. Close monitoring of liver function is recommended when the two drugs are used together. Complimentary, sequential use of acitretin and cyclosporine has been recommended. Cyclosporine is fast acting but can cause nephrotoxicity with long-term use; acitretin's action is slow in plaque psoriasis, but acitretin is not associated with cumulative toxicity. Thus, cyclosporine can be used initially to achieve rapid control over the psoriasis, followed by transition to acitretin to maintain safe long-term control. Both drugs can elevate triglyceride and cholesterol levels.

Side Effects

At low doses of acitretin (less than 25 mg per day), side effects are less common, and adverse effects generally occur at doses of 25 mg or more per day. Most patients will experience some side effects at the beginning of their treatment period. During this initiation period, the most commonly reported adverse effects include chelitis, alopecia, and peeling (Table 1); acitretin is, like isotretinoin, an oral retinoid, and the side effects of treatment are similar to those of isotretinoin (though acitretin has a longer half life requiring much longer pregnancy prevention). These effects are often reversible or subside with adjustment of dosage or cessation of treatment, though some patients who get severe alopecia may never want to take the drug again. Avoiding high doses can help reduce side effects. In addition, patients should be regularly monitored for elevations in liver enzymes, cholesterol, and triglycerides; in the past, screening for skeletal changes was recommended but this does not appear necessary in adults being treated for psoriasis (Table 4). The National Psoriasis Foundation's Systemic Treatment brochure (http://www.psoriasis.org/Document.Doc?id=161) is a wonderful resource for educating patients about the risks of and alternatives to acitretin treatment.

Table 2. Side effects of Acitretin

Common side effects	Chelitis
	Alopecia
	Skin dryness and peeling
	Headache
	Nose bleeds
	Nail Dystrophy
	Pruritus
	Nausea
	Diarrhea
Rare side effects	Depression
	Diffuse idiopathic skeletal hyperostosis (in young children on high dose treatment of xeroderma pigmentosa)
	Pancreatitis
	Leukopenia
	Toxic hepatitis (but not cirrhosis)
	Myopathy
	Pseudotumor cerebri
	Reduced night vision
	Retinoic acid syndrome
Teratogenicity may also occur without adherence to proper contraception	

Contraindications

Due to the teratogenicity of acitretin and potential for toxicity, there are some contraindications (Table 3). Absolute contraindications include severe liver failure, severe kidney failure, allergy to drug components, and pregnancy. Acitretin is classified as pregnancy category X due to retinoid embryopathy resulting in craniofacial dysmorphias, hip malformations, and spinal cord abnormalities; given the many alternatives now available, acitretin should not be used in women of child-bearing potential. In the rare case in which acitretin were used in such a patient, 2 effective forms of contraception should begin at least 1 month prior to initiation of treatment and continue use *for at least 3 years* after cessation of treatment because of the drug's long half-life. Patients on acitretin should be cautioned not to donate blood because of this teratogenic risk. Additional relative contraindications to the use of acitretin include hypercholesterolemia, bone abnormalities, leukopenia, and age under 14 years.

While some guidelines caution against using in patients with alcohol consumption, use in these patients may be appropriate. There is a risk of hepatotoxicity with alcohol and with acitretin, but patients can be monitored for that by checking liver function tests at 3 month intervals. There is also concern that the combination of acitretin plus alcohol can lead to esterification of the acitretin to etretinate; etretinate has a much longer half life. But as long as acitretin is not used in women of child-bearing potential, the potential conversion to etretinate caused by concurrent use of alcohol may be of no clinical significance.

Table 3. Patients eligible to use Acitretin

Inclusion Criteria	*Exclusion Criteria*
Extensive disease	Pregnancy
Very frequent recurrence	Breastfeeding
Impact on quality of life	Liver Failure or use hepatotoxic drugs
Poor control with topical treatment	Patient does not have severe renal failure or use nephrotoxic drugs
Failure to control psoriasis with other therapy	Patient has uncontrolled hyperlipidemia
Patient is over the age of 14	Child bearing potential
Patient does not have severe bone abnormalities	

Monitoring

Prior to starting a patient on acitretin, obtain a medical history and perform a baseline workup, including baseline liver function tests and lipid panel (Table 4). Educate patients of the most common side effects of the drug and preventative measures, as unexpected adverse effects can lead to poor adherence to treatment. Patients should be apprised of their other treatment options (the National Psoriasis Foundation Systemic Treatment brochure available at http://www.psoriasis.org/Document.Doc?id=161 is helpful in this regard).

Tips and Tricks

1. Encourage your patients to review The National Psoriasis Foundation's Systemic Treatment brochure (http://www.psoriasis.org/Document.Doc?id=161).

2. The appearance of chelitis is a useful sign that the correct bioavailability of acitretin has been reached.

3. The effects of ultraviolet radiation are enhanced by retinoids; thus, patients should avoid excessive exposure to sun lamps or sunlight.

4. When adding acitretin after initiation of phototherapy, reduce phototherapy dose by 50% one week prior to introducing acitretin (10 to 25 mg/d) to avoid sudden phototoxcity; gradually increase phototherapy dose according to phototoxicity and clinical response.

5. Radiological studies (i.e. targeted x-rays) are not warranted in acitretin therapy unless atypical musculoskeletal pain develops.

6. Patients with diabetes, obesity, and alcoholism can be monitored more frequently due to increased risk of hypertriglyceridemia and hepatotoxicity.

7. Acitretin is a potent teratogen and should not be used in women of child-bearing potential. If acitretin use is required by a woman of child-bearing potential, note that acitretin may reduce the efficacy of progestogen contraceptives (i.e. mini pill); choose a combined contraceptive pill with both estrogen and progestogen.

8. Ideally, for women of child bearing potential, pick another treatment that isn't teratogenic. If acitretin has to be used in women of

childbearing age in which pregnancy has been excluded, therapy with acitretin should be started on the second or third day of the next menstrual cycle once pregnancy has been excluded.

Suggested References

1) Haushalter K, Murad EJ, Dabade TS, Rowell R, Pearce DJ, Feldman SR. Efficacy of low-dose acitretin in the treatment of psoriasis. *J Dermatolog Treat.* 2011; 2:86-89.

2) Berbis P, Geiger JM, Vaisse C, Rognin C, Privat Y. Benefit of progressively increasing doses during the initial treatment with acitretin in psoriasis. *Dermatologica.* 1989; 178:88-92.

3) Gollnick HP, Dummler U. Retinoids. *Clin Dermatol.* 1997; 15:799-810.

4) Murray HE, Anhalt AW, Lessard R, Schacter RK, Ross JB, Stewart WD, et al. A 12-month treatment of severe psoriasis with acitretin: Results of a Canadian open multicentre trial. *J Am Acad Dermatol.* 1991; 24:598-602.

5) Ormerod AD, Campalani E, Goodfield MD. British Association of Dermatologists guidelines on the efficacy and use of acitretin in dermatology. *Br J Dermatol.* 2010; 162: 952-963.

6) Imcke E, Ruszczak Z, Mayer-da Silva Aet al. Cultivation of human dermal microvascular endothelial cells in vitro: immunocytochemical and ultrastructural characterization and effect of treatment with three synthetic retinoids. *Arch Dermatol Res.* 1991; 283:149–57.

7) Nijsten TE, Stern RS. Oral retinoid use reduces cutaneous squamous cell carcinoma risk in patients with psoriasis treated with psoralen-UVA: a nested cohort study. *J Am Acad Dermatol.* 2003; 49:644–50.

8) Iest J, Boer J. Combined treatment of psoriasis with acitretin and UVB phototherapy compared with acitretin alone and UVB alone. *Br J Dermatol.* 1989; 120:665–70

9) Kampitak T, Asawanonda P. The efficacy of combination treatment with narrowband UVB (TL-01) and acitretin vs narrowband UVB alone in plaque-type psoriasis: a retrospective study. *J Med Assoc Thai.* 2006; 89(Suppl. 3):S20–4.

10) Ozdemir M, Engin B, Baysal I et al. A randomized comparison of acitretin–narrow-band TL-01 phototherapy and acitretin–psoralen plus ultraviolet A for psoriasis. *Acta Derm Venereol (Stockh).* 2008; 88:589–9.

11) Mork NJ, Kolbenstvedt A, Austad J. Efficacy and skeletal side effects of 2 years acitretin treatment. *Acta Derm Venereol (Stockh).* 1992;72:445–8.

12) Rim JH, Park JY, Choe YB, et al. The efficacy of calcipotriol + acitretin combination therapy for psoriasis: comparison with acitretin monotherapy. *Am J Clin Dermatol.* 2003; 4(7):507–10.

13) Ruzicka T, Sommerburg C, Braun-Falco O, et al. Efficiency of acitretin in combination with UV-B in the treatment of severe psoriasis. *Arch Dermatol* 126(4):482–6 (1990 Apr).

14) Carretero G, Ribera M., Belinchon I, Carrascosa JM, Puig LI, Ferrandiz C, et al. Guidelines for the Use of Acitretin in Psoriasis. *Actas Dermosifiliogr.* 2013; 104(7):598-616.

15) Naldi L, Griffiths CEM. Traditional therapies in the management of moderate to severe chronic plaque psoriasis: an assessment of the benefits and risks. *Br J Dermatol.* 2005;152:597-615.

16) Searles AD, Lee AD, Feldman SR. Is concomitant use of methotrexate and oral retinoids dangerous? A review of the data regarding this combination. *J Am Acad Dermatol.* 2011 Apr;64(4):791-3.

17) Koo J. Systemic sequential therapy of psoriasis: a new paradigm for improved therapeutic results. J Am Acad Dermatol. 1999 Sep;41(3 Pt 2):S25-8.

18) Lee E, Koo J. Single-center retrospective study of long-term use of low-dose acitretin (Soriatane) for psoriasis. *J Dermatolog Treat*. 2004 Jan;15(1):8-13. PubMed PMID: 14754643.

19) Halverstam CP, Zeichner J, Lebwohl M. Lack of significant skeletal changes after long-term, low-dose retinoid therapy: case report and review of the literature. J *Cutan Med Surg*. 2006 Nov-Dec;10(6):291-9. Review. PubMed PMID: 17241599.

Table 4. Acitretin recommended monitoring and protocol checklist monitoring

1.	**Pregnancy screening and Contraceptive Use**	
A.	Women of childbearing age must undergo a pregnancy test within 2 weeks prior to therapy to exclude pregnancy	
B.	Effective contraception must be practiced 1 month prior to initiation of treatment and continued for 3 years after treatment has ceased	
2.	**Assess renal function**	
A.	Order urea, electrolytes, and creatinine	
	Prior to treatment	
3.	**Assess liver function**	
A.	Order LFTs (ASTs and ALTs), alkaline phosphatase, and bilirubin	
	Prior to treatment	
	At appropriate intervals, monthly monitoring for the first 3 months, then every 3-6 months thereafter	
4.	**Hyperlipidemia screening**	
A.	Order fasting serum cholesterol, triglycerides, HDL, and LDL	
	Prior to treatment	
	At appropriate intervals, monthly monitoring until lipids are stable, then every 3-6 months thereafter	
5.	**Abnormal glucose tolerance screening**	
A.	Order fasting glucose prior to treatment	
6.	**Hematologic disorder screening (optional)**	
	Order CBC and CMP prior to treatment	

Chapter 9: Cyclosporine

Leah Cardwell, Kathryn L. Anderson, Steven R. Feldman

Introduction

Cyclosporine is an immunosuppressive polypeptide used to prevent graft versus host disease in stem cell transplant recipients and prevent graft rejection in solid organ transplant recipients. In addition, cyclosporine is used in the treatment of immune-mediated diseases, including psoriasis and rheumatoid arthritis. Cyclosporine, via interaction with calcineurin, reduces production of IL-2 and other cytokines produced by T-lymphocytes. Cyclosporine is roughly as effective as methotrexate, but faster acting and with greater risk of long-term renal side effects. Thus, cyclosporine should be considered for acute, short-term treatment of severe psoriasis and when other systemic medications have failed. Safety and efficacy of cyclosporine can be improved through education and adherence to strict periodic monitoring guidelines.

Mechanism of Action

Cyclosporine is a lipophilic cyclic peptide composed of 11 amino acids. The drug binds with high affinity to cyclophilins (a family of cytoplasmic proteins). This drug-receptor complex competitively inhibits calcineurin. Ultimately, the drug inhibits the translocation of NF-AT leading to decreased transcriptional activation of cytokine genes for IL-2, IL-3, IL-4, TNF-alpha, CD40L, GM-CSF, and IFN-gamma and reduction in lymphocyte proliferation. Cyclosporine specifically affects T-helper lymphocytes, T-suppressor lymphocytes, and T-cytotoxic lymphocytes.

Dosing

Cyclosporine may be administered via various formulations including oral, intravenous, topical and ophthalmic. However, the intravenous form is only used in extenuating circumstances due to increased risk of toxicity. Oral bioavailability of the drug is limited due to inadequate absorption, metabolism by enzymes in the bowel mucosa, and first-pass effect in the liver. Cyclosporine is metabolized in the gut mucosa to a minimal extent, and extensively by CYP-450 in the liver with excretion in the bile. Bile salts are necessary for the absorption of cyclosporine. Absorption may be increased with consumption of a fatty meal at the time of drug administration.

Development of microemulsion oral formulations allows absorption of the drug in the absence of bile salts and leads to increased drug bioavailability. Therefore the microemulsion formulation is generally preferred, particularly in individuals with biliary diversion or cholestasis. Initial dosing of cyclosporine for psoriasis is 2.5-4 mg/kg divided into two doses, sometimes somewhat higher for short periods to get rapid control of flaring psoriasis.

Efficacy

A meta-analysis of several randomized studies involving patients with severe psoriasis determined that after 10-12 weeks of cyclosporine treatment at 1.25, 2.5, and 5 mg/kg/day, there were PASI reductions of 44.4%, 69.8% and 71.5% respectively. In a study which assessed severe psoriasis patients assigned to either a 2.5 mg/kg/day starting dose and an increasing regimen or a 5.0 mg/kg/day starting dose and a decreasing regimen, PASI 50 response rates at 12 weeks was similar for both groups while PASI 75 response rates at 12 weeks was higher in the step-down regimen group.

Side Effects

Frequency and severity of side effects are less in patients using the drug for treatment of dermatological and autoimmune disorders versus usage in transplant recipients due to lower doses and more flexibility in decreasing medications if signs of side effects arise. Nevertheless, the side effects of cyclosporine, particularly effects on renal function, limit its use (Table 1). In some cases, side effects associated with cyclosporine may be reversible upon discontinuation of use.

Table 1. Side effects of Cyclosporine

Nephrotoxicity Acute increase in creatinine Secondary to vascular dysfunction and tubular dysfunction Rarely Hemolytic Uremic Syndrome
Hypertension Due to renal vasoconstriction and sodium retention
Gingival hyperplasia Due to fibrous hyperplasia Reported in 30% of patients
Neurotoxicity Manifests with symptoms such as headaches, tremors, seizures, psychosis, paresthesias Often normalizes with discontinuation of use
Bone Loss Due to increased bone turnover
Electrolyte and Lab Abnormalities Hyperkalemia, hypomagnesemia, and/or hyperuricemia
Malignancy Squamous cell skin cancer Benign or malignant lymphoproliferative disorders Via production of TGF-beta Function of drug dose and duration of use
Cutaneous Abnormalities Hirsutism, epidermal cysts, acne, folliculitis, keratosis pilaris and sebaceous hyperplasia Due to modulation of protein kinase C expression in hair epithelial cells→promotes proliferation of hair epithelial cells
Gastrointestinal effects Nausea, vomiting, diarrhea and discomfort Rare increased liver enzymes
Infections Incidence may be reduced through proper vaccination adherence
Hyperlipidemia/Hypertriglyceridemia Often normalizes with discontinuation of drug

Contraindications

Patient should be screened to ensure that they meet eligibility for cyclosporine use (Table 2). Absolute contraindications to use of cyclosporine include malignancy, uncontrolled hypertension, renal insufficiency, uncontrolled infection, immune deficiency, high cumulative dose of previous psoralen and UVA light phototherapy, cutaneous T-cell lymphoma, and hypersensitivity to cyclosporine. Due to the immunosuppressive effects of cyclosporine, it is prudent to inquire about the presence of these contraindications in a patient being considered for cyclosporine therapy.

Monitoring

There are various recommended monitoring guidelines to assist healthcare providers in monitoring for potential side effects of cyclosporine therapy (Table 3). At each office visit, patients should be asked questions pertaining to common side effects of cyclosporine use. Malignancy screening guideline includes colonoscopy, mammogram, pap smear, etc. Due to the gingival hyperplasia side effect, patients on cyclosporine should be instructed to visit the dentist at 6-month intervals. Age-appropriate vaccinations should be obtained prior to starting cyclosporine therapy, and pneumococcal and killed influenza vaccinations should be administered annually.

Tips and Tricks:

1. The use of cyclosporine should be limited to short time periods where a quick improvement in severe psoriasis is necessary.

2. Avoid using cyclosporine for more than two years, as this increases the chance of kidney failure. Biologic medications are much safer options in patients with severe disease necessitating systemic treatment.

Suggested References

1) Yoon HS, Youn JI. A comparison of two cyclosporine dosage regimens for the treatment of severe psoriasis. *J Dermatolog Treatment.* 2007; 18(5):286-90.

2) Colombo MD, Cassano N, Bellia G, Vena GA. Cyclosporine regimens in plaque psoriasis: an overview with special emphasis on dose, duration, and old and new treatment approaches. *Scientific World Journal.* 2013.

Table 2. Cyclosporine: Checklist for Patient Eligibility

Patient has no current malignancy and consideration paid to history of previous malignancy	
Patient is not breastfeeding	
Patient does not have uncontrolled hypertension	
Patient does not have renal insufficiency	
Patient is not immunosuppressed	
Patient does not have an active or chronic infection	
Patient has not received a high cumulative dose of psoralen and UVA light phototherapy	
Patient has no history of lymphoproliferative disease, including lymphoma	
Patient has no history of hypersensitivity to cyclosporine	
Patient has exhausted other more conventional therapies (ie. Topical steroids, topical retinoids, Vitamin D analogues, etc.)	

Table 3. Monitoring checklist for cyclosporine

1.	**Skin exam**	
	Assess for actinic damage, skin malignancies, herpes simplex, and viral warts	
2.	**Assess kidney function**	
	Take blood pressure, and blood tests for serum creatinine, blood urea nitrogen, and glomerular filtration rate	
	Urinalysis	
	Baseline, repeat every other week for 2 months, and then monthly if stable	
	After 1 year or continuous therapy	
3.	**Assess for electrolyte abnormalities**	
	Perform a blood test for potassium, magnesium, and uric acid levels	
	Baseline, then monthly. Frequency can be reduced once stable levels are obtained.	
4.	**Assess for lipid abnormalities**	
	Perform a blood test for fasting lipids	
	Baseline, then monthly. Frequency can be reduced once stable levels are obtained.	

Chapter 10: Apremilast

Sara Moradi Tuchayi

Introduction

Despite the large number of therapeutic agents currently available for psoriasis, patients' desire for a safe, oral medication—one with fewer side effects than methotrexate—has been elusive. A step in that direction was made with the approval of apremilast (Otezla®) for psoriasis and psoriatic arthritis.

Mechanism of Action

Apremilast is a specific inhibitor of phosphodiesterase-4 (PDE4) enzyme. PDE inhibitors should not be unfamiliar. The most widely used drug in humans, caffeine, is a non-specific PDE inhibitor. PDE inhibitors prevent the breakdown of cyclic AMP, raising intracellular cyclic AMP levels and reducing production of multiple cytokines.

Unlike widely used biologics, being a small molecule, apremilast can be taken orally. PDE4 is the critical phosphodiesterase enzyme in inflammatory cells, and therefore PDE4 inhibitors can be effective as anti-inflammatory drugs with few side effects.

Dosing

The standard dosing of apremilast is 30mg twice a day. In order to improve tolerability and prevent diarrhea with the initiation of treatment, consider introducing the drug gradually (Table 1). Celgene, apremilast's manufacturer, provides convenient bubble packaged sample kits that make a gradually increasing starting dose more convenient.

Table 1. Apremilast dosing to help prevent diarrhea

Day	Dosage
Day 1	10 mg in the morning
Day 2	10 mg in the morning and 10 mg in the evening
Day 3	10 mg in the morning and 20 mg in the evening
Day 4	20 mg in the morning and 20 mg in the evening
Day 5	20 mg in the morning and 30 mg in the evening
Day 6 and on	30 mg twice daily

In patients with severe renal impairment (creatinine clearance <30 m L/minute), dose adjustment should be considered; starting with 10 mg in the morning on days 1 to 3 and then titrating to 20 mg on days 4 and 5. Maintenance dose with severe renal impairment is 30 mg once daily in the morning starting on day 6.

There is no need to reduce the dose in patients with hepatic failure. Using apremilast with CYP450 enzyme inducers (such as rifampin, phenobarbital, carbamazepine, phenytoin) is not recommended, but there are no significant drug-drug interactions with oral contraceptives, ketoconazole or methotrexate.

Efficacy

In a phase III study of apremilast for moderate-to-severe psoriasis, 33.1% of patients achieved 75% reduction in Psoriasis Area and Severity Index (PASI75) after 16 weeks of treatment. Apremilast's efficacy is less than that of biologics, less than that of perhaps half the usual dose of etanercept (PASI75 of ~40%)[1] and far less than the effectiveness of the usual doses of adalimumab or ustekinumab, which offer PASI75 rates of about 67% to 70%.

Apremilast can be a good therapeutic choice for moderate-to-severe psoriasis patients for patients who are willing to consider a medication that seems very safe but which does not result in the great majority of patients having a rip roaring good response to treatment. It may be a good choice for patients unable to take methotrexate or for patients who did not see satisfying results from methotrexate and who do not wish to begin an injectable biologic treatment. Apremilast's wholesale price is less than biologics but more than $20,000/year, and that may be a hurdle for some patients.

Side Effects

The most common observed distinctive side effect is diarrhea, seen in roughly 8-15% of patients. Other side effects include nausea, vomiting, weight loss, headache, and upper respiratory tract infection. Rarer side effects include gastroesophageal reflux disease, hypersensitivity, migraine, and suicidal ideation. In order to decrease the risk of diarrhea and other common side effects, gradual dose increase is recommended.

No cases of tuberculosis or lymphoma were reported through week 16. There was no apparent increased risk of serious opportunistic infection. In case of severe side effects discontinuation of therapy should be considered.

Although the side effects are not as severe as the potential side effects of methotrexate, they could have the potential to reduce patients' adherence. Common side effects of apremilast tend to fade over time and mostly resolve after 15 days of treatment, so efforts should be made to encourage patients to develop a habit of taking this medication through this period and beyond. Due to lack of studies in pregnant women apremilast is considered Pregnancy Category C. Apremilast should only be used in pregnant or breastfeeding women if the potential benefit justifies the potential risk (see Chapter 15).

Monitoring

Weight monitoring is recommended as modest weight loss is seen in some patients (something many patients might consider a benefit of the drug). Discontinuation of therapy should be considered in case of significant weight loss. Renal function should also be assessed. Patients should be monitored mood changes, depression, and suicidal thoughts during therapy.

Tips and Tricks

1. Use the startup packs to help minimize the risk of diarrhea. Developing diarrhea late in therapy is unusual.

2. Adherence is usually worse in clinical practice than in clinical studies. That could limit the effectiveness of apremilast, which isn't the most effective drug to begin with. Help patients develop a plan to assure good adherence.

3. If patients are worried about the drug, let them know that caffeine is also a phosphodiesterase inhibitor.

4. Apremilast should only be used in pregnant or breastfeeding women if the potential benefit justifies the potential risk.

5. Some patients may find the possible weight loss side effect to be a positive attribute about the drug.

6. Consider dosage reduction in patients with severe renal impairment (creatinine clearance <30 mL/minute).

7. No laboratory monitoring is required for patients on apremilast.

78

Suggested References:

1) Signorovitch JE, Betts KA, Yan YS, et al. Comparative efficacy of biologic treatments for moderate to severe psoriasis: a network meta-analysis adjusting for cross-trial differences in reference arm response. *Br J Dermatol.* 2014.

Table 2. Apremilast Checklist

Provide patients with information about side effects and how soon to expect improvement.	
Monitor weight regularly during therapy.	
Use with caution in patients with a history of depression or suicidal thoughts. Ask patients about these symptoms during therapy.	
Ensure patients are not on CYP450 enzyme inducers (such as rifampin, phenobarbital, carbamazepine, and phenytoin).	
Schedule follow up appointment in 2-4 weeks following the prescription of apremilast to assess for response and potential side effects (see Chapter 4 on adherence for advice on how to assure good adherence to treatment)	

Chapter 11: Use of Biologics for Psoriasis

Alexandria Bass, Michael E. Farhangian, and Steven R. Feldman

Introduction

Biologic medications for psoriasis, or "biologics," are a class of systemic medications that target specific portions of the body's immune system (Figure 1). They are complex glycoproteins made in living organisms and are given via injection or by intravenous infusion. Unlike other systemic medications, such as methotrexate and cyclosporine, biologics are used to target a specific part of the immune system, usually either a soluble protein or cell surface receptor. Because they are highly specific for targets that have relatively narrow functions in the immune system, biologics are safer than some of the older systemic medications used to treat psoriasis.

For psoriasis and/or psoriatic arthritis treatment, biologics target a variety of proteins that all play a vital role in the development of psoriasis. One such protein is tumor necrosis factor-alpha (TNF-alpha), which is involved in mediating the inflammatory cascade. Medications that block this protein are called TNF-alpha inhibitors. Examples are adalimumab (Humira), infliximab (Remicade®), etanercept (Enbrel®), and two newer medications indicated for psoriatic arthtritis, certolizumab pegol (Cimzia®) and golimumab (Simponi®). Another family of medication, called interleukin inhibitors, inhibit other chemical messengers involved in the inflammatory cascade. Ustekinumab (Stelara®) targets interleukin 12 (IL-12) and interleukin 23 (IL-23). Secukinumab (Cosentyx®), ixekizumab (in clinical trials), and brodalumab (in clinical trials) target interleukin 17 (IL-17) (Figure 1, Table 1).

80

Figure 1. Biologics for treating psoriasis and/or psoriatic arthritis

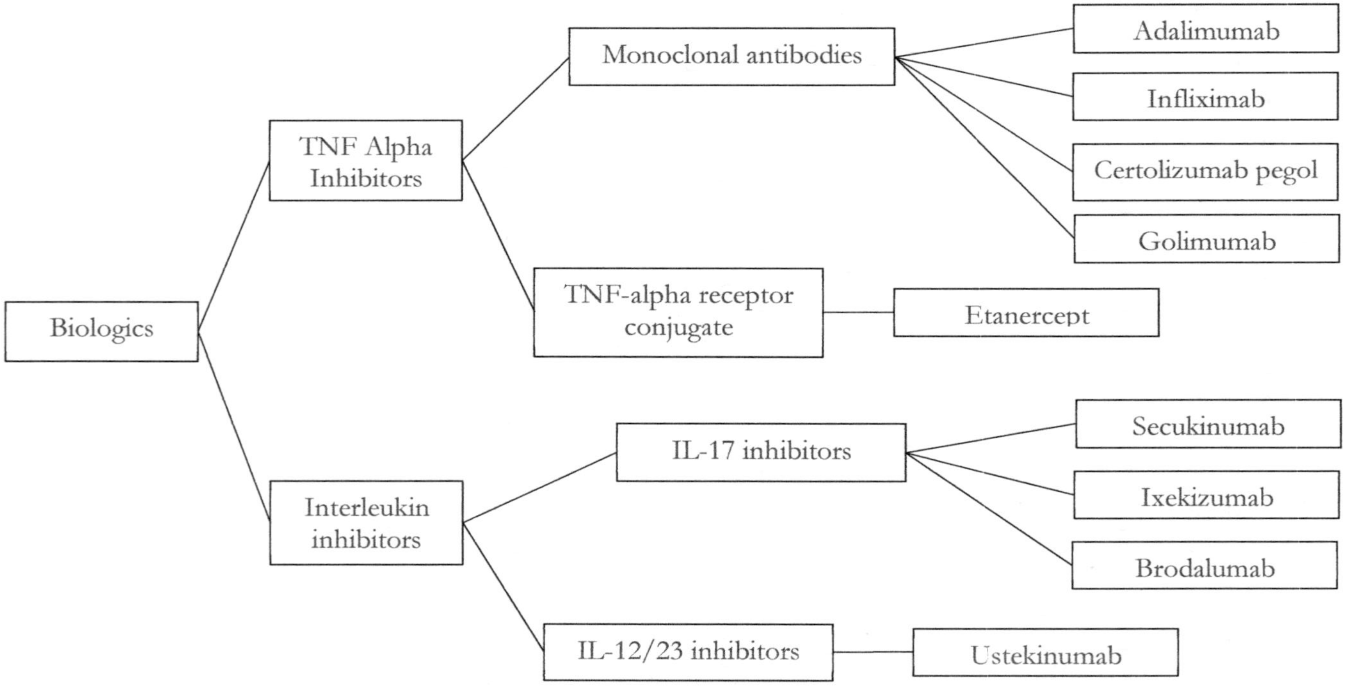

Table 1. Pharmacokinetics and dosing for FDA approved biologics (as of May 2015) used for psoriasis

Medication	Route of Administration	Initial Dosing	Maintenance Dosing	Half-Life	Bioavailability
TNF-alpha inhibitors					
Adalimumab (Humira®)	Subcutaneous	Week 0: 80 mg	Week 1 and then every 2 weeks: 40 mg	10-20 days	64%
Infliximab (Remicade®)	Intravenous	Week 0, 2, and 6: 5 mg/kg	Every 8 weeks: 5 mg/kg	8-9.5 days	100%
Etanercept (Enbrel®)	Subcutaneous	1st 12 weeks: 50 mg twice per week	50 mg weekly	80 hrs	76%
Certolizumab pegol (Cimzia®)	Subcutaneous	Weeks 0, 2, and 4: 400 mg (2 separate 200 mg syringes)	Every 2 weeks: 200 mg (can be increased to 400 mg monthly, once clinical response has been noted)	14 days	76%-88%
Golimumab (Simponi®)	Subcutaneous	Monthly: 50 mg injection monthly	Monthly: 50 mg injection (can be increased to 100 mg)	12 ± 3 days	51%
Interleukin Inhibitors					
Ustekinumab (Stelara®)	Subcutaneous	Week 0 and 4: 45 mg (≤ 220 lbs) 90 mg (≥ 220 lbs)	Every 12 weeks: 45 mg (≤ 220 lbs) 90 mg (≥ 220 lbs)	15-32 days	57.2%
Secukinumab (Cosentyx®)	Subcutaneous	Week 0-4: 300 mg weekly (2 separate 150 mg injections)	300 mg every 4 weeks	22-31 days	55%-77%

Indications

Biologics are recommended for patients with moderate-to-severe psoriasis (or psoriatic arthritis, Table 2). They are a great alternative to those who could not tolerate other systemic medications due to side effects, as well those who have failed other treatments such as methotrexate, cyclosporine, and/or phototherapy. Choosing which biologic to prescribe depends on the patient, their disorder, and their preferences (and often what their insurance company will pay for). There is not one perfect biologic for every patient. Issues such as cost, efficacy, convenience, and tolerability are all factors that need consideration. Infliximab is given by intravenously infusion over several hours, while others can be given subcutaneously. All of the biologics discussed are effective for psoriasis and/or psoriatic arthritis.

There are many potential strategies physicians can use when starting biologics. One approach is to start with a weaker medication allowing opportunity to switch to a stronger medication if needed; an alternative is to start with the medication that is least costly for the patient. Perhaps it is best to start with the medication the patient is most comfortable with using. Physicians may prescribe other medications in conjunction with biologics, such as methotrexate, which helps prevent antibody formation and increase efficacy. Also, the medications used for psoriasis can be combined with topical therapies for resistant plaques.

Table 2. Indications for biologics

Medication	Psoriasis	Psoriatic Arthritis
TNF-alpha inhibitors		
Adalimumab	✓	✓
Infliximab	✓	✓
Etanercept	✓	✓
Certolizumab		✓
Golimumab		✓
IL-12/23 inhibitor		
Ustekinumab	✓	✓
IL-17 inhibitors		
Secukinumab	✓	Effective in trials
Ixekizumab	In Phase II of clinical trials	
Brodalumab	In Phase II of clinical trials	

Side effects

The main concern with biologic treatment is the risk of infection, since biologics work by inhibiting immune function; however the risk of serious infections is low. Most infections reported in patients on biologics are usually mild upper respiratory infections, but serious infections—such as tuberculosis or systemic fungal infections—may occur (though perhaps no more often than with placebo). Another common side effect is injection reactions, but they are usually mild and subside without discontinuing the medication. Some more serious, but uncommon side effects, specific to TNF-alpha inhibitors are development or activation of a demyelinating disorder, such as multiple sclerosis, exacerbation of Hepatitis B infection, exacerbation of congestive heart failure, or a hematologic disease, such as aplastic anemia, thrombocytopenia, and leukopenia. Although these adverse effects are rare, the benefits of using biologics in patients with moderate-to-severe psoriasis outweigh the risk.

Contraindications

Due to the (at least theoretical) immunosuppressive nature of biologics, they should be used with caution in people who already have a weakened immune system. Also, biologics should not be started in people with infections such as untreated latent or active tuberculosis, other active infections, or people who recently received a live vaccine. Some biologics, such as TNF-alpha inhibitors, have additional contraindications and should be used in caution in people with a multiple sclerosis or a first degree relative with multiple sclerosis, people with hepatitis B infection, and people with New York Heart Association Class 3 or 4 congestive heart failure.

Adherence to biologics

Poor adherence to medication is a common problem, even with biologics. Although the dosing of biologics is not as tedious as topical therapies, there is still a significant amount of non-adherence, leading to suboptimal clinical results. Since the medication will not work in patients who don't use them, methods to encourage good adherence in patients should be employed for best possible clinical outcomes. Establishing a strong, trusting physician-patient relationship, educating the patient, office visits, reminders, calendars, and/or correlating treatment with a particular weekly task may all be effective methods to increase adherence in patients.

Getting your patient started on a biologic

Biologics are costly and may be difficult to afford for some individuals. However, between insurance, manufacturer copayment assistance programs and foundation support, most patients are able to access these treatments. The average wholesale price (AWP) of these biologics (Table 3) represent prices that most patients do not see. Given the contracting and rebates that are in place between insurers and drug manufacturers, health care providers probably never know what the true cost of the drug is to the patient's insurer.

Table 3. TNF-alpha inhibitor costs

TNF-alpha inhibitor	Amount of medication	Average Wholesale Price (AWP) (November 2014)
Infliximab	100mg in 20 mL vial	$1,113.89
Enbrel	50mg/mL x 4 syringes	$3,496.99
	25mg/0.5mL x 4 syringes	$1,748.50
Adalimumab	40mg/0.8mL prefilled syringe x 2 syringes	$3,496.37
	Starter Pack 40mg/0.8mL x 4 syringes	$6,992.72
Certolizumab pegol	400mg/2mL prefilled syringe	$3,322.98
Golimumab	50mg/0.5mL x 1 syringe	$3,574.69

Most insurance coverage will require prior authorizations showing that the provider has tried at least one alternative, less expensive option before the insurer will cover the cost of a biologic. The paperwork generally requires basic patient information, body surface area affected, previous therapies used, and assurance that tuberculosis testing has been done. This process of getting patients approved for treatment with biologics is extensive, but the effort will hopefully pay off since biologics are generally very effective in treating psoriasis. Third party assistance to get the approval may be obtained from specialty pharmacies and through programs set up by drug manufacturers.

There are many patient assistance programs available to help your patient with paying for their medication if needed. If your patient is uninsured, has Medicare or Medicaid, or has insurance but cannot afford the cost of their medications, they may be eligible for financial assistance from the manufacturing company or an outside foundation. On the National Psoriasis Foundation website, there is a list of contacts for specific medications, the manufacturer, and phone number. This information can be found at http://www.psoriasis.org/access-care/insurance/financial-assistance/biologics. Patient assistance foundations, such as The Assistance Fund, Patient Advocate Foundation, Chronic Disease Fund, and Patient Access Network Foundation, can also assist with payment of medications. These can be found on the National Psoriasis Foundation website at http://www.psoriasis.org/access-care/insurance/financial-assistance/copay.

Choosing the "Right" Biologic

Deciding which biologic to use for psoriasis is complicated. Factors to consider include efficacy, safety, comorbidities, cost, and preference for dosing regimen and delivery method.

All biologics are effective, some more than others. Of the biologics currently approved for psoriasis (as of May 2015), secukinumab is the most effective biologic, with 82% of individuals experiencing PASI 75 12 weeks after starting therapy. Next, in decreasing order of effectiveness is infliximab (80% achieving PASI 75), adalimumab (70% achieving PASI 75) and ustekinumab (67% achieving PASI 75), and etanercept (49% achieving PASI 75).

For psoriatic arthritis, there are variances in effectiveness as well. Generally, TNF inhibitors seem to have an edge in effectiveness over other options (though the comparison with IL-17 inhibitors is not yet clear).

Clinical results for biologics can be assessed around 3 months; if no significant benefit is observed by then, a different approach should be considered. Patients who did not achieve clinical success with one biologic may still respond to another because these medications act using different mechanisms of action and because some poor response is due to specific anti-drug antibodies. Methotrexate can be given in conjunction with many biologics in order to increase efficacy and to help prevent antibody formation.

Chapter 12: Tumor Necrosis Factor-alpha (TNF-alpha) Inhibitors

Alexandria Bass, Michael E. Farhangian and Steven R. Feldman

Introduction

TNF-alpha is a cytokine involved in the inflammatory cascade that was initially discovered in cancer research. It mediates growth factors and cytokines that cause hyperproliferation of the epidermis in patients with psoriasis. In patients with psoriasis, TNF-alpha levels in the skin and joints are elevated, leading indirectly to rapid growth of keratinocytes in the epidermis and to inflammation in the skin and joints. The level of TNF-alpha in the body correlates with disease severity. TNF-alpha inhibitors (Table 1) block this inflammatory cytokine, thereby decreasing inflammation and improving clinical severity. All TNF-alpha inhibitors, with the exception of certolizumab and golimumab (which are approved only for psoriatic arthritis treatment), are indicated for use in patients with moderate to severe plaque psoriasis and psoriatic arthritis. Due to the costliness and insurance hurdles, TNF inhibitors are generally prescribed when at least one non-biologic systemic treatment has failed. The three TNF-alpha inhibitors most widely used for psoriasis are adalimumab, infliximab, and etanercept.

Mechanism of Action

Adalimumab, infliximab, and etanercept all block TNF-alpha and are indicated for psoriasis and psoriatic arthritis; however they vary in their chemical composition and the ways in which they target TNF-alpha. Adalimumab and infliximab are monoclonal antibodies against TNF-alpha. They both bind to membrane bound and soluble TNF-alpha, thereby neutralizing its activity. On the other hand, etanercept is a receptor fusion protein that is made up of two human TNF alpha receptors fused to the Fc portion of a human antibody, allowing it to have a longer half-life in the body than naturally occurring soluble TNF receptors. Etanercept acts through competitive inhibition as a receptor decoy to bind free TNF-alpha, decreasing TNF activity (Table 1).

Dosing

TNF-alpha inhibitors are all administered via subcutaneous injection with the exception of infliximab, which must be delivered intravenously. Patients can be trained to self-administer biologics that are delivered via subcutaneous injections. However, patients treated with infliximab must travel to a physician's office or infusion center to have the medication administered, making it a less convenient treatment option for most patients. The protocols for dosing TNF-alpha inhibitors vary (see Chapter 11 on biologics). TNF inhibitors tend to work best if they are used continuously, rather than being stopped and restarted, particularly in the case of infliximab. However, rapid, severe rebound of psoriasis usually does not occur when TNF inhibitors are discontinued.[1]

Efficacy

TNF-alpha inhibitors are all effective medications, with some more effective than others (see Chapter 11 for an overview of biologics). In short-term clinical trials of TNF inhibitors, infliximab was most effective for psoriasis treatment with 80% of patients seeing 75% improvement in Psoriasis Area and Severity Index (PASI75) after 3 months. Adalimumab closely followed with 70% of patients achieving a PASI75, and 49% attained a PASI75 with etanercept. In regards to psoriatic arthritis treatment, all three medications were near equally effective with about 40% achieving 50% improvement in the American College of Rheumatology (ACR) score used to measure the severity of arthritis. Clinical results can be assessed at 3 months; if no significant benefit is observed by then, a different approach should be considered.

Patients who do not achieve clinical success with one TNF inhibitor may still respond to another. For example, a patient may be started initially on the least potent TNF inhibitor, etanercept, for their psoriasis. This allows for the option to prescribe a more effective medication, such as adalimumab in the future, if the patient does not see adequate improvement with etanercept. On the other hand, if a patient is started on adalimumab, and no clinical response is noticed, they may have developed anti-adalimumab antibodies, in which case etanercept could still be effective for this patient.

---

[1] Rebound on discontinuation has been thought to be a characteristic of psoriasis treatments, but it may be a characteristic of patients. While rebound does not typically occur with TNF-alpha inhibitors, it may be because most of the patients treated with TNF-alpha inhibitors do not have rapid rebound on discontinuation. Some may, however.

Sometimes, methotrexate is given in conjunction with TNF-alpha inhibitors to increase efficacy and to help prevent antibody formation. Although there is no consensus on what dose of methotrexate would be adequate in these patients, 7.5mg per week might be a good starting point. Antibodies form most commonly to infliximab and less so to adalimumab; etanercept appears to induce little antibody response of any significance. Infliximab has the highest rate of decreased effectiveness over time, perhaps because it has a murine component, leading to higher antibody formation. Infliximab given on a regular basis and in combination with methotrexate appears to improve safety and reduce loss of efficacy. Deciding which TNF-alpha inhibitor to initiate treatment requires collaboration between you and your patient. Considering cost, convenience, disease severity, and contraindications are all factors to be discussed with your patient in choosing the best therapy for their psoriasis.

New TNF-alpha Inhibitors

Certolizumab (Cimzia®) and golimumab (Simponi®) are other TNF-alpha inhibitors that were FDA approved for the treatment of psoriatic arthritis in 2008 and 2009, respectively. They are very similar to the other TNF-alpha inhibitors; however, there are slight differences. Not as much research has been performed with these medications in psoriasis as there has been with the other TNF-alpha inhibitors (Table 1).

Table 1. TNF-alpha inhibitors mechanism of action and dosing schedule

TNF-alpha inhibitor	Mechanism of Action	Route	Dosing	Combination
Adalimumab	Human monoclonal antibody	Subcutaneous	Initially (week 0): 80 mg Week 1 and then every 2 weeks: 40 mg	-Methotrexate -Phototherapy -Topical treatments - NSAIDS
Infliximab	Human/murine monoclonal antibody	Intravenous	Week 0, 2, 6, and then every 8: 5 mg/kg	-Methotrexate **Do not use with:** -Phototherapy (may increase the risk of skin cancer)
Etanercept	Receptor decoy	Subcutaneous	1st 12 weeks: 50 mg twice per week Maintenance: 50 mg weekly	-Methotrexate -Phototherapy -Topical treatments -NSAIDS
Certolizumab pegol	Humanized monoclonal PEGylated antibody (the antibody is combined with polyethylene glycol (PEG) to extend its half-life)	Subcutaneous	Weeks 0, 2, and 4: 400 mg (2 separate 200 mg syringes) Maintenance: 200 mg every 2 weeks (can be increased to 400 mg monthly, once clinical response is noted)	-Methotrexate (Indicated to be used with methotrexate but can be used alone if needed)
Golimumab	Human monoclonal antibody	Subcutaneous	50 mg injection monthly (can be increased to 100 mg)	-Methotrexate

Side Effects

The side effects of these medications are similar (Table 2). In regards to viral hepatitis, TNF inhibitors can exacerbate hepatitis B infection. TNF-alpha normally suppresses hepatitis B viral replication, so if inhibited, viral replication increases, and the disease can be reactivated. Conversely, TNF-alpha inhibitors may help control hepatitis C virus infection.

Although a number of common side effects were reported in clinical trials of TNF inhibitors, for the majority, there was no significant difference appreciated between the TNF-alpha inhibitor and control groups.

Table 2. Side effects of TNF-alpha inhibitors

Common side effects	Increases risk of infections (especially upper respiratory tract infections)
	Painful, burning, or itching injection site reactions (especially with etanercept)
	Exacerbation of congestive heart failure
	Medication interactions
Rare side effects	Developing or reactivating tuberculosis
	Developing or exacerbating a demyelinating disorder
	Drug induced lupus
	Viral hepatitis (usually Hepatitis B)
	Liver injury (hepatocellular or autoimmune injury)
	Hematologic disease (such as aplastic anemia, isolated leukopenia, and thrombocytopenia)
	Increased risk of cancer (such as lymphoma and skin cancer due to immunosuppression; the increased risk of lymphoma may be due to the disease and not to the drug)

Contraindications

Due to the immunosuppressive nature of TNF-alpha inhibitors, there are some contraindications (Table 3). People at risk for infection (for example people with recurrent chest infections or indwelling catheter), malignancy (except for treated non-melanoma skin cancer), and those with active or untreated latent tuberculosis are not recommended to use TNF-alpha inhibitors. Also, those with demyelinating disorders or congestive heart failure are advised not to use this class of medications. TNF-alpha inhibitors are classified as pregnancy category B so they should be used with caution in pregnant and nursing women. TNF inhibitors are approved for other indications in children (etanercept and adalimumab are approved down to age 2 for juvenile arthritis) and may be used for children with psoriasis, though caution should be used when initiating off label treatment in the pediatric population.

Monitoring

Due to the side effects of TNF-alpha inhibitors, such as tuberculosis, hepatitis, basal and squamous cell skin cancer, and hematologic issues, there are some recommended screening and tests to be performed in patients using these medications (Table 4).

Tips and Tricks

1. Concomitant treatment with low dose methotrexate can be used to augment and prolong treatment efficacy and can also prevent antibody formation against TNF alpha inhibitors.

2. If patients on etanercept experience a flare after their loading dose, consider either continuing the higher loading dose if covered by insurer, adding topicals/phototherapy/or oral agent, or switching to a different drug altogether.

Frequently Asked Questions (FAQs)
Will TNF-alpha inhibitors cure my psoriasis and/or psoriatic arthritis?

- These medications will NOT cure the disorder; however they will alleviate most symptoms and decrease damage to joints in those with psoriatic arthritis. Continuous usage of these medications is the best way to prevent recurrence of symptoms.

What is my risk of encountering a serious side effect, such as infection, multiple sclerosis, and/or lymphoma?

- Many patients and providers commonly worry about the potential side effects of TNF-alpha inhibitors, making providers less inclined to prescribe these medications. All the TNF-alpha inhibitors have been associated with rare cases of all of the side effects listed, such as infections, multiple sclerosis, and lymphoma. However, patient's taking TNF-alpha inhibitors have a lower lifetime risk of acquiring an infection (such as tuberculosis), lymphoma, or other neurological diseases as the general public.[1] Typically, infections are encountered as the most frequent side effect, but the risk is still only <0.1%.[2] The benefits of biologics may outweigh the risks for patients with moderate-to-severe psoriasis.

What are ways to decrease adverse reactions?

- Most mild, common adverse reactions seem to resolve with further usage of the medications. Methods to reduce some of the common side effects such as injection or infusion reactions are rotating the injection area or slowing the infusion rate. Stopping the medication if the patient develops a fever, and carefully reviewing the contraindications and checklist discussed above before initiating treatment are other ways to reduce adverse effects.

---

[1] Kaminska E, Patel I, Dabade TS, Chang J, Qureshi AA, O'Neill JL, Balkrishnan R, Feldman SR. Comparing the lifetime risks of TNF-alpha inhibitor use to common benchmarks of risk. *J Dermatolog Treat*. 2013 Apr;24(2):101-6.

[2] Burmester GR, Panaccione R, Gordon KB, McIlraith MJ, Lacerda AP. Adalimumab: long-term safety in 23 458 patients from global clinical trials in rheumatoid arthritis, juvenile idiopathic arthritis, ankylosing spondylitis, psoriatic arthritis, psoriasis and Crohn's disease. *Ann Rheum Dis*. 2013 Apr;72(4):517-24.

Table 3. Checklist for Patients eligible to use TNF-alpha inhibitors

Patient is not immunosuppressed	
Patient does not have active or untreated latent tuberculosis	
Patient does not have an active or chronic infection (including HIV, Hepatitis, indwelling urinary catheters, chronic leg ulcers)	
Patient is not pregnant	
Patient does not have moderate or severe congestive heart failure	
Patient does not have a personal or family history of demyelinating diseases, including multiple sclerosis	
Patient does not have a hematologic disorder	
Patient does not have a lymphoproliferative disease, including lymphoma	
Patient does not have melanoma or solid organ cancer	
Patient has exhausted other less expensive systemic options	

Table 4. TNF-alpha inhibitor monitoring checklist

1.	**Tuberculosis screening**	
A.	Test for tuberculosis using either a PPD skin test or QuantiFERON TB Gold	
	Prior to treatment	
	At appropriate intervals, often performed yearly	
B.	If (+) for active or latent disease: 9 months of isoniazid therapy is recommended before starting treatment, however, length of treatment can be made on an individual basis	
2.	**Hepatitis B screening**	
A.	Order hepatitis B surface antigen, surface antibody, and core antigen prior to treatment	
B.	If (+) for active or chronic infection: treatment is postponed until the hepatitis is managed by a hepatologist	
3.	**Assess liver function (optional)**	
A.	Order LFTs (ASTs and ALTs)	
	Prior to treatment	
	At appropriate intervals, often evaluated at least yearly with periodic CMPs	
4.	**Vaccination**	
A.	Get patient up to date on vaccinations before starting the biologic	
B.	**Avoid live or live attenuated vaccines.** If a live vaccine needs to be administered, it is recommended to have one month between the vaccination and starting the medication.	
5.	**Hematologic disorder screening (optional)**	
A.	Order CBC and CMP	
	Prior to treatment	
	Every 3 months for the first year then twice a year	
6.	**Skin cancer screening (optional)**	
A.	Perform a total body skin exam	
	Prior to treatment	
	At appropriate intervals, usually performed yearly	

Chapter 13: Ustekinumab

Hossein Alinia, Michael E. Farhangian, and Steven R. Feldman

Introduction

Ustekinumab was approved by the European Medicines Agency (EMA) and the US Food and Drug Administration (FDA) in 2008 and 2009 respectively for treatment of moderate to severe plaque psoriasis in adult patients who are candidates for phototherapy or systemic therapy and the treatment of active psoriatic arthritis (PsA) in 2013. Ustekinumab is a first line biologic options and is also a good treatment choice in patients who have previously failed treatment with a TNF-alpha antagonist due to its different mechanism of action.

Mechanism of Action

Ustekinumab is a monoclonal antibody against interleukins 12 and 23, preventing them from binding to their receptor expressed on the surface of immune cells and inhibiting the downstream inflammatory signaling pathways. Pathways activated by IL-12 and IL-23 are linked to the pathogenesis of psoriasis by activation of natural killer (NK) cells and T-cell (CD4+) differentiation. It may be helpful to tell patients that IL-12 and IL-23 are overexpressed in psoriatic lesions, and the goal is to bring them down to normal levels.

While ustekinumab was designed as an IL12-blocker, its effects on IL-23 are likely critical to its efficacy. Three of the genes that are linked to psoriasis are IL-23-related genes. This can also help reassure patients that the ustekinumab treatment may be targeting the specific problem causing the psoriasis.

Dosing

Ustekinumab is administered by subcutaneous injection. After a single baseline dose, patients should take the second dose at week 4 followed by injection of the same dose every 12 weeks. The recommended dose for psoriatic arthritis is the same as plaque psoriasis, which is 45mg for patients who are under 100kg (approximately 220 pounds), and 90mg for patients who weigh more than 100kg. If there is excellent improvement in psoriasis that wears off before the next 12 week dose is due, consideration may be given to treating every 8 or 10 weeks (as opposed to every 12 weeks) or to increasing dose to 90 mg (in patients receiving 45mg dose). If no response is observed after 28 weeks, ustekinumab is not likely to be effective and should be discontinued.

The patient's body weight and the levels of antibodies against ustekinumab affect the medication's pharmacokinetic properties. Although the impact that anti-drug antibodies have in ustekinumab is not entirely elucidated, it has been associated with decreased serum levels and poor therapeutic response in some patients.

Efficacy

Patients achieve PASI75 in 78% of cases treated with 90mg of ustekinumab at week 28. Efficacy with ustekinumab was maintained for up to 3 years and PASI75 with ustekinumab 45 mg and 90 mg are 63% and 72%, respectively. For patients weighing more than 100 kg, the PASI75 response rate is about 20% higher with 90mg dose than in the 45 mg dose. By contrast, for lighter patients (≤100 kg), PASI 75 response rates are similar between the 90mg and 45mg dose. Ustekinumab has an ACR 20 response of about 50%, ACR 50 response of about 28% and ACR 70 of about 14% at week 24 of treatment for psoriatic arthritis. Ustekinumab is also indicated for treatment of enthesitis and dactylitis.

Side effects

Ustekinumab is quite safe, and may be associated with lower serious adverse event (AE) rates and lower rates of infections compared to the TNF antagonists (Table 1). So far, the long-term safety outcomes are unaffected by the dose of ustekinumab or the cumulative exposure to the drug. Overall AE rates, rates of AEs leading to discontinuation, and rates of overall infections decreased over time from Year 1 to Year 5.

Table 1. Adverse events

More common adverse events	Less common adverse events
Nasopharyngitis	Cellulitis
Upper respiratory tract infection	Herpes zoster
Headache	Diverticulitis
Fatigue	Injection site reactions (pain, swelling, pruritus, induration, hemorrhage, bruising, and irritation)
Diarrhea	
Back pain	
Dizziness	One reported case of reversible posterior leukoencephalopathy syndrome (RPLS), a non-infectious process
Pharyngolaryngeal pain	

*Adverse event rates were comparable with placebo

Since ustekinumab affects the immune system, it *may* increase the risk of serious bacterial, fungal, and viral infections, although clinical trial data so far show lower infection rates with ustekinumab than with placebo. Caution should be taken for patients with chronic infections, history of recurrent infection, or with conditions that predispose them to infections (diabetes or residence/travel from areas of endemic mycoses). Ustekinumab should not be administered to patients with active infection (including TB) until it is adequately treated (Table 2). Patients with latent TB should initiate treatment for TB prior to starting ustekinumab. In worldwide trials, 167 patients with latent TB were initiated on anti-tuberculous treatment and were started on ustekinumab; none developed reactivation of TB. Patients should be evaluated for active TB during and after treatment.

Because ustekinumab affects the immune system, it may, in theory, increase the risk of malignancy (though so far there has been no detectable increased malignancy risk identified). The rapid appearance of multiple cutaneous squamous cell carcinomas has been reported in patients who had pre-existing risk factors for developing non-melanoma skin cancer. Having more than 60 years of age, medical history of prolonged immunosuppressant therapy and PUVA treatment may increase this risk. Sunbeds and sunbathing should be avoided (unless needed as a form of phototherapy) to reduce the risk of skin cancer.

The chance of serious hypersensitivity reactions is very low but hypersensitivity reactions may be serious like anaphylaxis or angioedema or just a rash and urticaria. Skin reactions may also occur such as pustular psoriasis and erythrodermic psoriasis.

One case of reversible posterior leukoencephalopathy syndrome (RPLS)— a very rare neurological disorder that can present with headache, seizures, confusion and visual disturbances—was reported in a patient on ustekinumab; it is not clear whether the RPLS was caused by ustekinumab. RPLS is not caused by demyelination or a known infectious agent but it might be fatal. Ustekinumab should be discontinued and supportive treatment should be started for RPLS.

The safety of ustekinumab in combination with other immunosuppressive agents or phototherapy has not been evaluated. In psoriatic arthritis studies, concomitant MTX use did not influence the safety and efficacy of ustekinumab.

Contraindications

As with all immunosuppressant medications, patients should not receive live vaccines during treatment with ustekinumab. Ustekinumab may diminish the therapeutic effect and increase the risk of infection and toxic effect of live vaccines, at least in theory, though no clear risk has been documented. To assure safety, live-attenuated vaccines should not be given for at least 3 months after ustekinumab therapy.

Ustekinumab is a pregnancy category B drug. The administration of high doses of ustekinumab to animal models during pregnancy and lactation had no adverse effects on females or fetuses and abortion rates were similar, with and without exposure to the drug (see Chapter 15 for more on treating psoriasis in pregnancy). Caution should be exercised when ustenkinumab is administered to women who are nursing. The unknown risks to the infant should be weighed against the known benefits of breast-feeding. Ustekinumab is expected to be excreted in the milk but whether this is clinically significant is unknown. There are families who are genetically deficient in IL-23; they exhibit sensitivity to BCG vaccination and atypical salmonella infections (problems not identified with ustekinumab treatment so far).

Monitoring

Due to the potential for side effects with ustekinumab, there are several recommended screening tests to perform in patients before and after they start ustekinumab (Table 3). Many of the recommended tests are optional; baseline tuberculosis testing is considered essential. Ustekinumab could normalize the formation of CYP450 enzymes. In patients who are receiving medications metabolized by CYP450 enzymes, monitoring for therapeutic effect (like warfarin) or drug concentration (like cyclosporine) should be considered.

Tips and tricks

1. Giving ustekinumab in the office assures good adherence to the treatment. Home administration is also an option.

2. If the drug works well for 8-10 weeks but the psoriasis starts coming back before the next 12 week dosing, other treatments (topical, photo or systemic) could be added, or the ustekinumab frequency can be increased to every 8-10 week dosing.

Suggested References

1) Wofford J, Menter A. Ustekinumab for the treatment of psoriatic arthritis. *Expert Rev Clin Immunol.* 2014 Feb;10(2):189-202.

2) Griffiths CE, Girolomoni G. Does p40-targeted therapy represent a significant evolution in the management of plaque psoriasis? *J Eur Acad Dermatol Venereol.* 2012 Aug;26 Suppl 5:2-8.

3) Scanlon JV, Exter BP, Steinberg M, Jarvis CI. Ustekinumab: treatment of adult moderate to-severe chronic plaque psoriasis. *Ann Pharmacother.* 2009 Sep;43(9):1456-65.

4) Cingoz O. Ustekinumab. MAbs. 2009 May-Jun;1(3):216-21.

5) Meng Y, Dongmei L, Yanbin P, Jinju F, Meile T, Binzhu L, Xiao H, Ping T, Jianmin L. Systematic review and meta-analysis of ustekinumab for moderate to severe psoriasis. *Clin Exp Dermatol.* 2014 Aug;39(6):696-707.

6) Weitz JE, Ritchlin CT. Ustekinumab : targeting the IL-17 pathway to improve outcomes in psoriatic arthritis. *Expert Opin Biol Ther.* 2014 Apr;14(4):515-26.

7) Chandler DJ, Bewley A. Ustekinumab for the treatment of psoriatic arthritis. *Expert Rev Clin Pharmacol.* 2014 Mar;7(2):111-21.

8) Kumar N, Narang K, Cressey BD, Gottlieb AB. Long-term safety of ustekinumab for psoriasis. *Expert Opin Drug Saf.* 2013 Sep;12(5):757-65.

9) Famenini S, Wu JJ. The efficacy of ustekinumab in psoriasis. *J Drugs Dermatol* 2013 Mar;12(3):317-20.

10) Wine-Lee L, Keller SC, Wilck MB, Gluckman SJ, Van Voorhees AS. From the Medical Board of the National Psoriasis Foundation: Vaccination in adult patients on systemic therapy for psoriasis. *J Am Acad Dermatol.* 2013 Dec;69(6):1003-13.

Table 2. Checklist for patients eligible to use ustekinumab

Patient is not immunosuppressed	
Patient does not have active or untreated latent tuberculosis	
Patient does not have an active infection	
Patient has failed topical therapy and other less expensive systemic medications	
Patient is not taking any contraindicated medication	
Patients did not receive BCG vaccine in the last year	
Patients did not receive live vaccine in the last 2 week	
Patients who have severe allergy to latex	

Table 3. Ustekinumab monitoring checklist

1.	**Tuberculosis screening**	
A.	Test for tuberculosis using either a PPD skin test or QuantiFERON TB Gold	
	Prior to treatment	
	At appropriate intervals, often performed yearly	
B.	If (+) for active or latent disease: 9 months of isoniazid therapy is recommended before starting treatment, however, length of treatment can be made on an individual basis	
2.	**Hepatitis B screening**	
A.	Order hepatitis B surface antigen, surface antibody, and core antigen prior to treatment	
B.	If (+) for active or chronic infection: treatment is postponed until the hepatitis is managed by a hepatologist	
3.	**Assess liver function (optional)**	
A.	Order LFTs (ASTs and ALTs)	
	Prior to treatment	
	At appropriate intervals, often evaluated at least yearly with periodic CMPs	
4.	**Vaccination**	
A.	Get patient up to date on vaccinations before starting the biologic	
B.	**Avoid live and live attenuated vaccines.**	
5.	**Hematologic disorder screening (optional)**	
A.	Order CBC and CMP	
	Prior to treatment	
	Every 3 months for the first year then twice a year	
6.	**Skin cancer screening (optional)**	
A.	Perform a total body skin exam	
	Prior to treatment	
	At appropriate intervals, usually performed yearly	
7.	**Side effects**	
A.	Discuss the warnings with patients: skin cancer, RPLS, injection reactions and infection.	
B.	Follow up for the patents with chronic infections, history of recurrent infection, or with conditions and recurrent infections	
C.	Screen for the presence of acute infection	

Chapter 14: Secukinumab

Leonora Culp, Michael E. Farhangian, and Steven R. Feldman

Introduction

Although there are many systemic agents approved for treatment of psoriasis, getting patients clear of their psoriasis is still a hurdle. Secukinumab is the newest approved biologic medication (as of April 2015) for the treatment of moderate to severe psoriasis. It functions as an inhibitor of interleukin-17 (IL-17). Two other inhibitors of IL-17, brodalumab and ixekizumab, are currently undergoing clinical trials, but have yet to be approved by the Food and Drug Administration for treatment of psoriasis. In general, IL-17 inhibitors have a high efficacy, fast onset, and few known side effects.

Mechanism of Action

Secukinumab is a monoclonal antibody that selectively binds and neutralizes interleukin 17A (IL-17A), a pro-inflammatory cytokine implicated in the pathogenesis of psoriasis. IL-17A is one of 7 subtypes of the IL-17 family and is produced by helper T-17 cells (Th17). By binding free IL-17A, secukinumab prevents it from binding to its receptor and subsequently inhibits inflammation and epidermal changes in psoriasis, including hyperkeratosis, acanthosis and parakeratosis. Secukinumab also maintains the integrity of the skin-barrier by preventing the down-regulation of filaggrin caused by IL-17A.

Dosing

The recommended dose for secukinumab is 300 mg by subcutaneous injection (given as 2 separate 1 mL injections of a 150 mg/mL formulation). It is administered weekly for the first 5 weeks and then once every 4 weeks thereafter. Secukinumab clearance is independent of the kidney and liver so no modification of the dose is needed for patients with renal or hepatic impairment.

Efficacy

Four phase III clinical trials have been conducted on secukinumab. PASI75 rates at 12 weeks averaged 75-87% and 67-87% for 300 and 150 mg secukinumab formulations. Modified IGA scores were between 62-73% and 51-53% for 300 and 150 mg secukinumab. PASI75 rates and modified IGA success rates are 10-20% higher for the 300mg compared with the 150 mg dose. Efficacy is higher with 300 mg compared to 150 mg independent of patient weight, so the 300 mg dose is recommended for all patients. Overdosage is unlikely, as doses of up to 3,000 mg have been given IV without serious side effects. One phase III clinical trial compared both concentrations of secukinumab to etanercept. Secukinumab 300 mg was better at clearing skin than etanercept (PASI75 rates of 77% for secukinumab 300 mg and 44% for etanercept 50 mg). In the CLEAR (**C**omparison to assess **L**ong-term **E**fficacy, s**A**fety and tole**R**ability of secukinumab vs. ustekinumab) trial, a head-to-head phase III trial comparing secukinumab to ustekinumab, secukinumab demonstrated superiority in achieving PASI 90 at week 16 (79.0% vs. 57.6%, P<0.0001) and PASI 75 at week 4 (44.3% vs. 28.4%, P<0.0001).

Side Effects

The most common side effects with secukinumab are increased risk of common mild infections, headache, eczema, pruritus and diarrhea (Table 1). Infections are more common during the 12 week induction period than the maintenance period. The mechanism for increased common infections is not well defined; it is possible that patients whose skin (and joint) disease has cleared spend more time in public and are simply exposed to more common infections.

There is an increased risk of candida infections with IL-17 inhibition, which is dose dependent. All candida infections in the secukinumab trials responded to standard treatment and did not necessitate drug discontinuation.

No systemic candidiasis infection, reactivation of latent tuberculosis (TB) or viral hepatitis were observed in any of the trials. While no cases of reactivated TB have been reported, screening for active and latent TB prior to starting secukinumab is recommended (Table 2).

Neutropenia is a rare side effect with secukinumab. The majority of cases of neutropenia were mild, transient, and reversible. Three cases of neutropenia were found in patients with non-serious infections including rhinitis, upper respiratory tract infections, and cystitis, though no cases resulted in drug discontinuation. As a precaution, a complete blood count should be performed if a patient on secukinumab presents with concerning symptoms or signs of infection.

With other biologics such as adalimumab, the formation of anti-drug antibodies (ADA's) could lead to a decrease in the efficacy of the drug. However, only 0.4% of patients in clinical trials developed ADA's to secukinumab. Furthermore, these antibodies did not lead to loss of efficacy or decreased drug concentration.

While a slight increase in serum transaminases was observed in patients on secukinumab, the majority of these cases were transient, resolving during the study. No cases of drug-induced liver injury were noted.

Secukinumab did not appear to increase the risk of solid tumors, lymphoma, leukemia, or skin cancer. Four patients developed malignant melanoma on secukinumab, but these individuals had several risk factors including prior exposure to phototherapy, TNF-alpha antagonist or methotrexate use.

Hypersensitivity reactions can occur with secukinumab. Urticaria was the most common reaction. All cases of urticaria were non-serious and mild to moderate in severity.

Table 1. Side effects of secukinumab

Most common minor side effects	Increases risk of infections (especially upper respiratory tract infections, nasopharyngitis, and mucocutaneous candidiasis)
	Headache
	Eczema
	Diarrhea
	Pruritus
Rare side effects	Exacerbation of Crohn's disease (about 1 in 1,000 in the clinical trials)
	Severe hypersensitivity reaction
	Anti-drug antibodies
	Neutropenia

Contraindications

Secukinumab should be used with caution in patients with Crohn's disease. In prior studies, secukinumab was not effective at treating Crohn's disease. In clinical trials for psoriasis, there were 3 patients who had flares of their Crohn's disease out of over 3,000 patients in those trials.

Live vaccines should not be given while on secukinumab (because there is no study showing they would be safe, not because they have been shown unsafe). If any live vaccines are needed, they should be given prior to initiating treatment with secukinumab. Nevertheless, a clinical study found no impact of secukinumab on antibody responses to killed influenza and meningococcal vaccinations.

Secukinumab is classified as pregnancy category B drug with no adverse effects on pregnancy in animal studies. There are no clinical trials of secukinumab in pregnant women. Secukinumab should only be used during pregnancy if the benefits outweigh the potential, unknown risks to the fetus. Since very little is known about the safety of secukinumab during pregnancy and nursing, caution should be exercised when prescribing secukinumab in these patients.

Monitoring

Due to the side effects of secukinumab, there are several recommended screening tests to perform in patients before and after they start secukinumab (Table 3). Since long term data is not available for secukinumab, there are also several optional recommendations to prevent possible unknown long term side effects.

Tips and Tricks

1. Ideal patients for secukinumab are those who have failed topical treatment, are interested in a biologic with the best chance at clearing their skin, and also are aware of the potential for possible, unforeseen long term side effects due to lack of long term studies.

2. Routine CBCs and PPD tests should be administered to patients on secukinumab to watch for development of neutropenia and TB.

3. Given the cost of this new drug, there are many opportunities available to help patients afford secukinumab. These options include a patient assistance foundation, a manufacturer's coupon for free doses, and a $0 copay plan.

4. Deficiencies in the IL-17 pathway are associated with susceptibility to superficial candida infections. Let patients know about the risk of yeast infection and that you can prescribe fluconazole if needed.

Suggested References

1) Blauvelt A, Prinz JC, Gottlieb AB et al. Secukinumab adminstration by pre-filled syringe: Efficacy, safety and usability results from a randomized controlled trial in psoriasis (FEATURE). *British J Dermatol.* 2015;172: 484-493.

2) Gooderham M, Posso-De Los Rios CJ, Rubio-Gomez, GA et al. Interleukin-17 (Il-17) inhibitors in the treatment of plaque psoriasis: A review. *Skin Therapy Lett.* 2015;20: 1-5.

3) Yamauchi PS, Bagel J. Next- generation biologics in the management of plaque psoriasis: A literature review of il-17 inhibition. *J Drugs Dermatol.* 2015; 14: 244-50.

4) Ohtsuki M, Morita A, ABE M et al. Secukinumab efficacy and safety in Japanese patients with moderate-to-severe plaque psoriasis: Subanalysis from ERASURE, a randomized, placebo-controlled, phase 3 study. *J Dermatol.* 2014; 41: 1039-1046.

5) Paul C, Lacour JP, Kreutzer K et al. Efficacy, safety and usability of secukinumab adminstration by autoinjector/pen in psoriasis: a randomized, controlled trial (JUNCTTURE). *J Eur Acad Dermatol Venereo*l. 2014; 22: 1-9.

6) M, McKreage K. Secukinumab: First global approval. *Drugs.* 2015; 75: 329-338.

7) Langley RG, Elewski BE, Lebwohl M et al. Secukinumab in plaque psoriasis-results of two phase 3 trials. N Engl J Med. 2014;371: 326-38.

8) Colombel JF, Sendid B, Jouault T et al. Secukinumab failure in Crohn's disease: The yeast connection? *Gut.* 2013; 62: 800-801.

Table 2. Checklist for patients eligible to use Secukinumab

Patient is not immunosuppressed	
Patient does not have active or untreated latent tuberculosis	
Patient does not have an active or chronic infection (including HIV, Hepatitis, indwelling urinary catheters, chronic leg ulcers)	
Patient is not pregnant or nursing	
Patient does not have active Crohn's disease	
Patient has failed topical therapy and other less expensive systemic medications	

Table 3. Secukinumab recommended monitoring and protocol checklist

1.	**Tuberculosis screening**	
A.	Test for tuberculosis using either a PPD skin test or QuantiFERON TB Gold	
	Prior to treatment	
	At appropriate intervals, often performed yearly	
B.	If (+) for active or latent disease: 9 months of isoniazid therapy is recommended before starting treatment, however, length of treatment can be made on an individual basis	
2.	**Vaccination**	
A.	Get patient up to date on vaccinations before starting secukinumab	
	Avoid live or live attenuated vaccines. If a live vaccine needs to be given, administer the vaccine at least one month prior to start the medication.	
3.	**Hematologic disorder screening (optional)**	
A.	Order CBC	
B.	At appropriate intervals, if concerned for infection and/or neutropenia	
4.	**Skin cancer screening (optional)**	
A.	Perform a total body skin exam	
	Prior to treatment	
	At appropriate intervals, usually performed yearly	

Chapter 15: Special Situations

Alyson Snyder, Michael E. Farhangian, and Steven R. Feldman

Introduction

This chapter describes the variations from the standard psoriasis algorithm for patients who are pregnant, Human Immunodeficiency Virus (HIV) positive, immunosuppressed, diagnosed with hepatitis, or children. When there is a coexistent infection, the treatment of psoriasis should first begin by controlling the underlying disease. In all situations, mild, localized psoriasis (that doesn't involve the palms or soles) is generally treated the same way as a healthy adult: with topical medications and/or localized UVB phototherapy, in addition to as attention to good adherence. Variations from the standard algorithm for treating moderate-to-severe psoriasis patients are required to avoid toxicity of systemic treatments in at risk populations (Figure 1). Our main focus will be how the standard algorithm of treatment changes in these susceptible populations. For more detailed information on the drug classes and individual drugs, please see their corresponding chapters.

Pregnancy

Since the average age of diagnosis of psoriasis is the mid-twenties, psoriasis during pregnancy is not an uncommon occurrence. The course of psoriasis during pregnancy can be unpredictable, but normal physiologic changes of maternal immune suppression often leads to improvement of psoriasis during pregnancy. Moderate to severe psoriasis in pregnant patients can lead to gestational complications like low birth weight or preterm delivery, but these risks also seem to increase with use of systemic medications. The biggest challenge in treating psoriasis in patients who are pregnant is balancing the benefits of the medicine verses the risk of harm to the fetus (Table 1 & Table 2). There has been limited research done in pregnant individuals due to ethical concerns.

UVB phototherapy is safe and is considered first line in pregnant patients with moderate-to-severe psoriasis. Topical corticosteroids and vitamin D analogues are generally safe in pregnancy but there has not been much research on their absorption. Coal tar should be used sparingly in pregnancy if at all because it is carcinogenic in animals, and one study reported one incidence of a lethal genetic syndrome in a fetus from a woman using coal tar. Psoralen is contraindicated and topical tazarotene is categorized as a pregnancy category X drug due to the theoretical risk of significant absorption.

Biologics, specifically the TNF-alpha inhibitors and ustekinumab, appear safe in pregnancy & breast feeding and are labeled as pregnancy category B in the United States (Table 1). Conclusions on safety are derived from animal studies and experience treating inflammatory bowel disease and inflammatory arthritis. Ustekinumab and secukinumab are newer biologics rated pregnancy category B, and are so new that we have little data about their safety in pregnancy. Very small amounts of biologics, presumed to be of negligible impact, have been isolated in the breast milk. All TNF-alpha inhibitors and ustekinumab, but much less with etanercept, cross the placenta and are found in higher concentrations in the infant than in the mother. Due to the placental transfer of medication to the fetus and potential immunocompromising effect of these drugs on the infant immune system, it is recommended to discontinue these medications by the late 2nd or 3rd trimester or to postpone live vaccines until the newborn is 6-7 months of age. Apremilast is a new biologic rated pregnancy category C and at this time needs more data to determine its safety profile in pregnant women (Figure 1). Cyclosporine is pregnancy category C and before biologics, it was more widely used and may still have a role for rapid relief of severe flares. There is a considerable amount of data on cyclosporine use in pregnancy from transplantation patients that have linked cyclosporine use to preterm labor and low birth weights.

Medications that should not be used in pregnant patients are methotrexate and acitretin (Table 1). Methotrexate is an abortifacient and teratogen that causes cardiac, skeletal and central nervous system abnormalities. Methotrexate is contraindicated while pregnant or nursing and stays in the body up to three months after discontinuation. Acitretin is highly teratogenic, leading to severe defects of the cardiovascular, skeletal, and central nervous systems. Pregnancy and nursing should be avoided while on and three years after discontinuation of acitretin. Tazarotene is in the same retinoid class as acitretin, but is a topical formulation. Despite being a topical medication, tazarotene is still listed as pregnancy category X due to its theoretical potential to cause the same serious birth defects as other retinoids.

Table 1. Pregnancy Category of Psoriasis Medications

B	C	X
Adalimumab	Psoralen oral & topical	Methotrexate
Etanercept	Topical tacrolimus & pimecrolimus	Acitretin
Infliximab	Topical corticosteroids	Topical tazarotene
Certolizumab pegol*	Topical anthralin	
Golimumab*	Coal tar	
Ustekinumab	Cyclosporine	
Secukinumab	Apremilast	

*Approved for psoriatic arthritis

Table 2. Description Pregnancy Categories in the United States

Pregnancy Category	Explanation
A	No risk to fetus: human studies.
B	No risk to fetus: animal reproductive studies, no human studies.
C	Unknown risk to fetus: animal studies have shown an adverse effect on the fetus, no human studies, benefits may outweigh the risks.
D	Evidence of risk to fetus: human, investigational, or marketing studies; benefits may outweigh the risks
X	Contraindicated: animal, human, investigational, or marketing studies show fetal abnormalities; risks outweigh the benefits

Tips & Tricks:

1. Methotrexate, acitretin and tazarotene are category X, contraindicated in women who are pregnant or planning to become pregnant.

2. Psoralen is contraindicated and limit coal tar use in pregnancy.

3. First line for moderate-severe psoriasis is UVB phototherapy.

4. Second line for moderate-severe psoriasis is TNF-alpha inhibitors, ustekinumab, apremilast, or cyclosporine.

5. Discontinue TNF-alpha inhibitors and ustekinumab if possible in the late 2nd or 3rd trimester.

Table 3. Pregnancy Checklist

Ask if currently pregnant or plans to become pregnant in patients of childbearing age	
Check urine pregnancy test and counsel on contraception in women of childbearing age before prescribing methotrexate. Acitretin simply should not be used in women who may become pregnant.	

Figure 1. Algorithm of how to treat pregnant patients with psoriasis

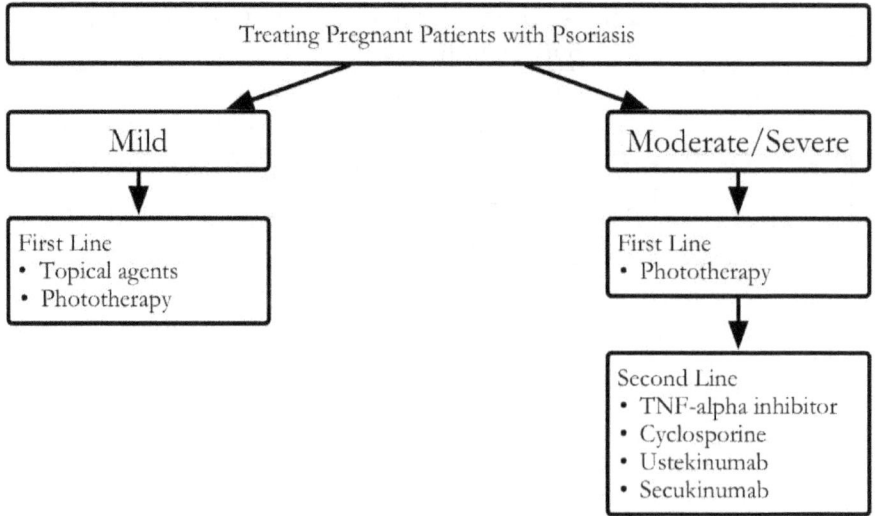

HIV & Immunosuppression

Although psoriasis is thought of as a disease of an over-active immune system, patients with a compromised, dysregulated immune systems may, paradoxically, present with psoriasis. Management of severe or resistant psoriasis in healthy adults often involves systemic medications such as methotrexate, cyclosporine and biologics that act directly on the immune system. These medications if used in a patient with a weakened immune system may predispose them to developing serious infections. UV phototherapy can be used cautiously; there may be some accelerated risk of skin cancer in immunosuppressed patients.

Oral retinoids such as acitretin can be a great choice if a systemic medication is needed, since retinoids provide benefit without significant immunosuppression. Patients who are immunosuppressed are often on multiple medications already, so the potential for interactions should be addressed in treatment planning. Hydroxyurea has been used in HIV treatment regimens and may be an appropriate systemic treatment choice for some patients. Dosing begins at 500 mg orally twice daily increasing by 500 mg daily increments every month up to 2 g daily. Complete blood count (CBC) should be monitored weekly after increasing dose and every 1-3 months while on a stable dose. Reports on the safety of biologics come mostly from case reports and so far do not find an increase in morbidity and mortality rates in HIV patients; TNF-inhibitors may improve some HIV symptoms as well as the psoriasis (Figure 2).

Tricks & Tips:

1. Systemic retinoids are a great choice for HIV and immunosuppressed patients

2. TNF-alpha inhibitors seem to be a safe option in patients with HIV or immunosuppression

Table 4. HIV & Immunosuppressed Checklist

Ensure that patients with HIV are being treated with HAART	
Do frequent skin checks in those patients using phototherapy	
Hydroxyurea monitoring: CBC weekly after increasing the dose and every 1-3 months while on a stable dose	

Figure 2. Algorithm of how to treat HIV positive patients with psoriasis

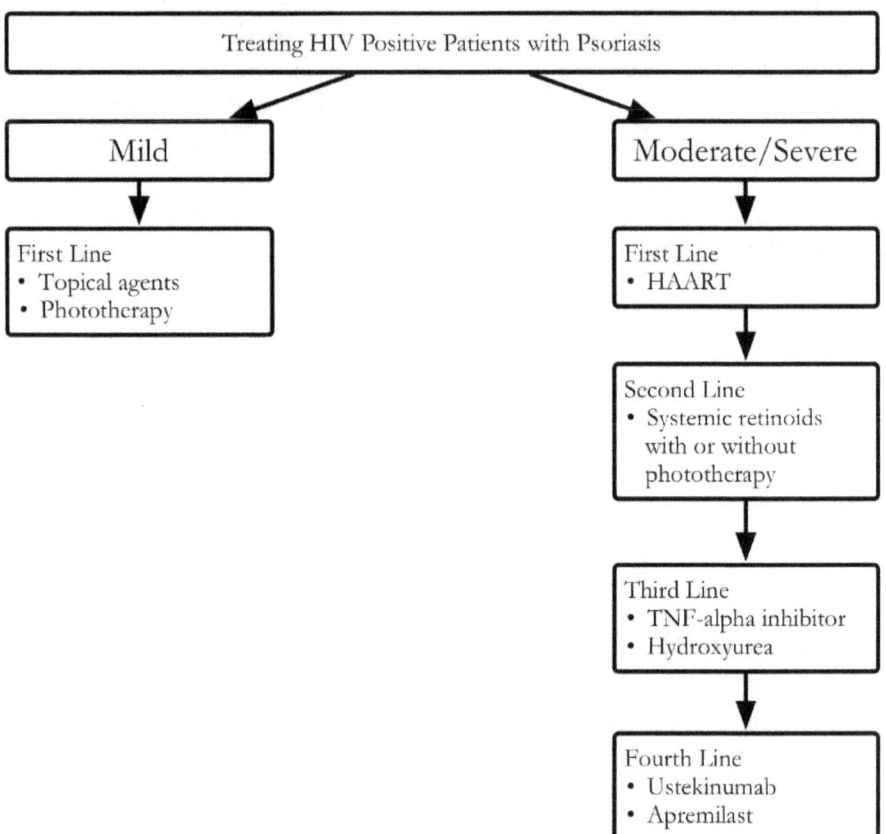

Hepatitis

Patients with hepatitis have restricted medication options and should be monitored to assure that treatments do not cause further liver damage or reactivation of the virus. Generally, medications that pose potential hepatotoxicity such as methotrexate, are relatively contraindicated.

Patients with hepatitis should have baseline liver function tests (LFT) and then follow up labs every 1-3 months. Before treatment with potentially hepatotoxic medications can commence, active hepatitis should be under control. Simultaneous treatment of hepatitis C virus with an appropriate antiviral to treat the hepatitis C and a TNF-alpha inhibitor for the psoriasis can be safe and effective in treating both diseases. Hepatitis B screening (for hepatitis B surface antigen [HBsAg] and anti-hepatitis B core antibody [anti-HBc]) should generally be done prior to initiating TNF-alpha inhibitors or ustekinumab due to the risk of reactivation of hepatitis B. HBsAg positive and possibly anti-HBc positive patients should be treated with appropriate hepatitis antivirals. Etanercept is currently the first line TNF-alpha inhibitor for treatment of psoriasis patients with chronic or a history of hepatitis B infection (Figure 3). When to perform a liver biopsy is controversial and ultimately up to a specialist, but may be indicated depending on disease state, lab values, cumulative medication dose, or amount of time on the medication. A hepatologist should be involved in the patient's care to treat active hepatitis, manage abnormal lab values, and/or perform a liver biopsy when indicated.

Tricks & Tips:
1. Etanercept is the first line TNF-alpha inhibitor for those with chronic or a history of hepatitis C

2. Consider referring to a hepatologist to manage patients' hepatitis

3. Consult a specialist regarding a liver biopsy

Table 5. Hepatitis Checklist

Check liver function tests at baseline and every 1-3 months in patients with liver disease or damage	
Control active hepatitis before starting treatment with a potentially hepatotoxic agent	
Check HBsAg & anti-HBc before starting a TNF-alpha inhibitor	

Figure 3. Algorithm of how to treat hepatitis patient with psoriasis

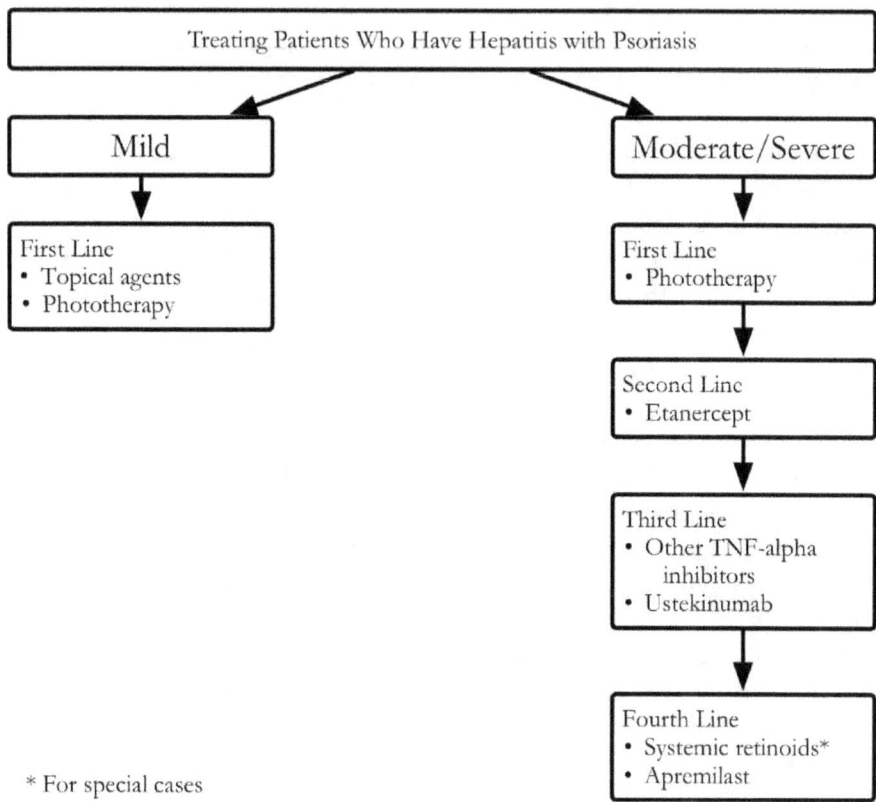

* For special cases

Alcoholism

Patients who drink alcohol excessively are at risk for exacerbations of their psoriasis. TNF-alpha inhibitors may help treat current liver damage in addition to psoriasis. Managing these patients can be particularly challenging because they may frequently miss appointments and may not be adherent with their treatment plans. Phototherapy may be a poor choice if patients are at risk of falling or cannot be relied on to use proper exposure times (Figure 4). Methotrexate may be contraindicated due to the greater risk of cirrhosis. Inquiry should be made about counseling, programs, or medications to help these patients quit consuming alcohol.

Tricks & Tips:

1. Alcohol cessation in those with alcohol misuse will lead to better outcomes in psoriasis treatment.

2. Methotrexate increases the risk of liver damage

3. Phototherapy may be a poor choice in patients with severe alcoholism

4. TNF-alpha inhibitors may be a good choice in patients with alcoholism

Table 6. Alcoholism Checklist

Counsel patients on the importance of alcohol cessation	
Be especially vigilant for adherence problems in patients with alcohol problems.	

Figure 4. Algorithm of how to treat alcoholics with psoriasis

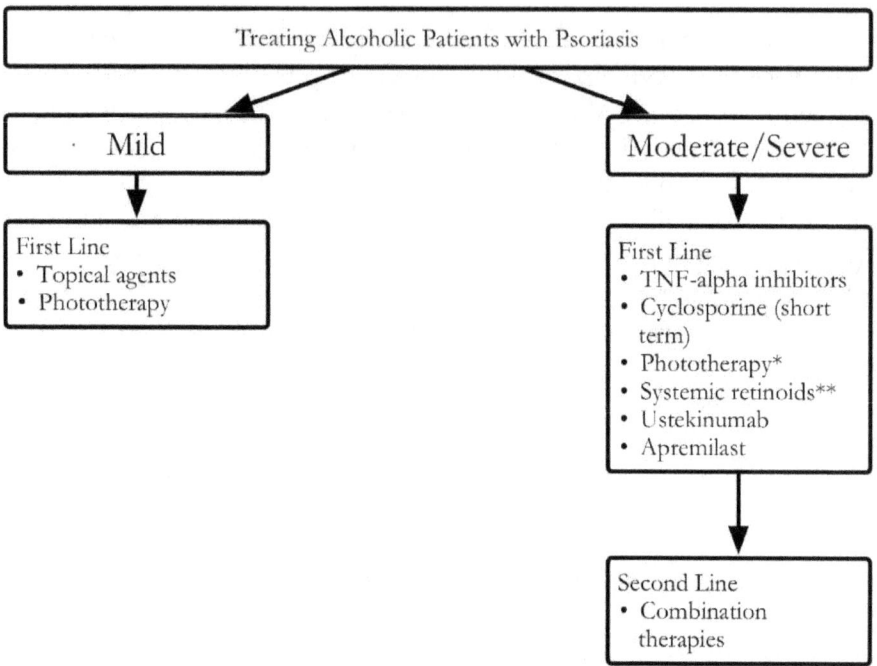

* Contraindicated if currently intoxicated

** For special cases

Children

Psoriasis is a devastating disease at any age, but can be extremely difficult for a child. Socially, bullying and embarrassment can ravage self-esteem. The treatment algorithm is very similar to that of an adult; mild disease treated with topical medications and/or UVB, and moderate to severe disease treated with phototherapy and systemic medications (Figure 5). The cumulative amount of UV should be monitored and limited to reduce the risk of developing skin cancers and photo aging later in life. Currently there is not a definition of the maximum safe dose of UV radiation, but the risk may be decreased by using UVB (even more so with narrow band UVB) instead of PUVA or natural light.

Most of the medications used for psoriasis have not been studied in the pediatric population, largely due to ethical reasons, and many are not approved by the FDA for this age group. For instance, while TNF-alpha inhibitors are approved as treatments for arthritis in young children, none of the TNF-alpha inhibitors are FDA-approved for psoriasis in children, and etanercept is the only TNF-alpha inhibitor to have a study done on pediatric patients. It is important to provide reassurance that although these medications are not FDA-approved for psoriasis in children, many of these drugs, such as methotrexate and TNF-alpha inhibitors, have been used to treat pediatric patients with psoriasis safely and effectively for years. (Table 7)

Table 7. Systemic medications used in the treatment of psoriasis and their level of evidence for the use in pediatrics

Systemic Medication	Level of Evidence
Adalimumab	Approved in 2 years or older for juvenile arthritis, 6 years or older for Crohn's disease
Infliximab	Approved for the treatment of Ulcerative colitis and Crohn's disease in children 6 years or older.
Etanercept	Approved as young as 2 years old for juvenile arthritis
Ustekinumab	One published case report of use in a 14 year old male with plaque psoriasis. A phase III multicenter randomized double-blind placebo-controlled trail evaluating efficacy and safety of adolescents with psoriasis is in progress outside the USA.
Apremilast	No trials or reports of use in pediatrics
Methotrexate	Approved in 2 years or older for juvenile rheumatoid arthritis and cancer chemotherapy. Pediatric use in many dermatologic and rheumatologic conditions
Cyclosporine	No adequate, well controlled studies in children. Pediatric use in many dermatologic and rheumatologic conditions in as young as 6 months old with similar side effects as adults.
Acitretin	No clinical trials. High-dose, long-term associated with bone abnormalities

Tips & Tricks

1. The treatment algorithm for children is similar to that of a healthy adult

2. First line treatment of moderate-severe psoriasis is phototherapy

3. Systemic medications can be used despite lack of FDA approval and testing

Table 8. Psoriasis in Children Checklist

Monitor cumulative UV therapy	

Figure 5. Algorithm of how to treat children with psoriasis

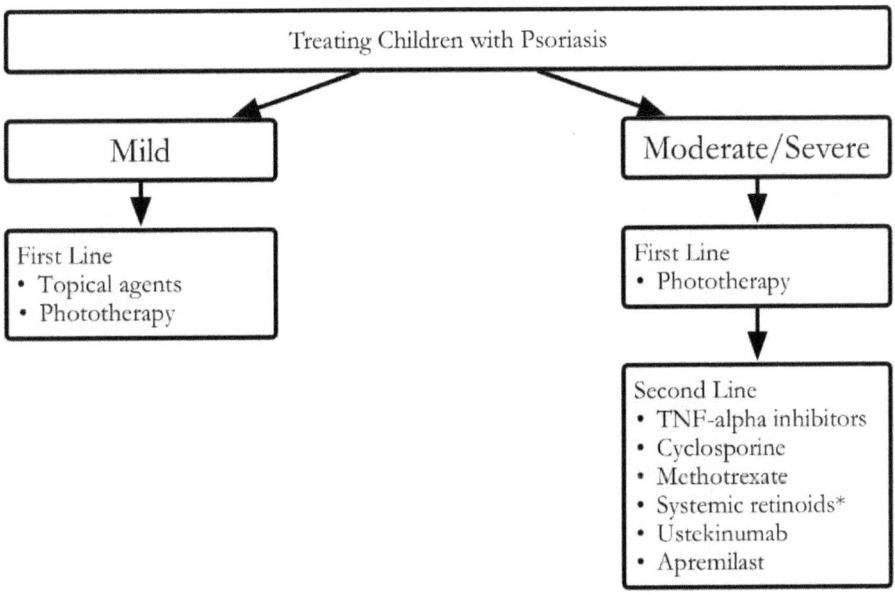

* For special cases

www.ingramcontent.com/pod-product-compliance
Lightning Source LLC
Chambersburg PA
CBHW070811180526
45168CB00002B/579